HOW CANCER CURED ME

Healing Brokenness and Disease

HOW CANCER CURED ME

Healing Brokenness and Disease

DAVID GIRA

Torchflame Books

Durham, NC

To the glory of God—
Father, Son, and Holy Spirit;

Amy, my beloved wife, friend,
and mother of my wonderful children—

Marcie, Hannah, and Caleb;

and the cancer community—
patients, survivors, loved ones,
and all who comfort and care.

Contents

Acknowledgments viii

Introduction x

Courage 1

Grace.. 13

Forgiveness 25

Compassion 37

Get-Up-And-Go 49

Strength.. 61

Faith.. 72

Provision 84

Patience 95

Rest 107

Trust.. 119

Joy 130

Friendship 143

Healing 154

Glory.. 165

Epilogue... 174

Endnotes 177

About the Author...................................... 178

Acknowledgments

Above all, thanks be to God, the Father of our Lord Jesus Christ. Thank you for giving me the mission to write this book. I hope it provides a faithful and fitting witness to the work you have done in my life and can do in the lives of others.

Amy, my beloved wife and soulmate, thank you for believing in this book and encouraging me to write it. Thank you for your love and patience with me throughout this process. Thank you for being with me and for me through cancer, with all its challenges. Together we have danced in the rain. May our story be a blessing to many others.

To my children, Marcie, Hannah, and Caleb, for believing in me. I hope this book will remind you always of how much I love you. I hope it will tell you of all God has done in our lives and can do in your life no matter what might one day be broken and in need of healing.

To my mom and dad, who brought me into this world and have loved me every day since. Thank you, Mom, for encouraging me to write about my cancer experience and for believing in me as a writer. Thank you, Dad, for teaching me about hard work, doing your best, and determination to complete the job.

Thanks to Jane Clark Moorman, my long-time counselor, and friend. You have been a healer for me at the deepest level. God has used you to bring healing to my soul and into many dimensions of my life. I would not possess the self-awareness required to write this book without you.

I am thankful for Dr. Jeffrey Crawford, Dr. Christopher Kelsey, and all the physicians, nurses, and staff at the Duke Cancer Clinic, for their expert and compassionate care.

I'm grateful for each church I have belonged to and served, to all my brothers and sisters in Christ, to my faithful friends, and especially to those who supported me through my cancer journey. You have shown me God's love. I have leaned on you and learned from you.

To my friends at Torchflame Books: Betty, Wally, and Elizabeth, thank you for believing in my book and its message, and thank you for encouraging me. Thank you to my editor, Meghan Bowker, for helping me sculpt, polish, and cull.

Introduction

My cancer diagnosis turned my world upside down. I experienced fear and every other emotion you would expect. All I wanted was to be physically healed. I wanted the cancer to be gone. Many prayed with me that I would be cured.

Physical healing began to happen quickly and in amazing ways. We watched in wonder the miracles of God and marvels of modern medicine collaborating to conquer cancer. My journey toward physical healing had many ups and downs, twists and turns, advances and setbacks. All these only made my story more inspiring and amazing. In less than two years, I went from stage four lung cancer to my first cancer-free report.

My physical healing amazed me and many others, but I sensed from the start that God wanted to do more than just physically heal me. God wanted to use my cancer to heal all the brokenness in my life. By the time I received my cancer-free report, twenty-two months after my diagnosis, my entire life had been changed for the better. In fact, cancer continued changing me in many positive ways even after it was gone. In countless ways, as crazy as it sounds, I am grateful for having had cancer.

I journaled daily starting September 1, 2017, the day my doctor diagnosed me with stage four lung cancer. My mother thought it would help me and probably others. You should always listen to your mom.

Several months later, I discovered a common theme running through all my writings; namely, God using my cancer to cure me. With that epiphany, God gave me a vision for this book and a title, and *How Cancer Cured Me* was born. More than clever and catchy, it was undeniably true, and I felt called by God to write it.

The Bible testifies, "And we know that in all things God works for the good of those who love him, who have been called according to his purpose" (Romans 8:28). Admittedly, when it comes to bad things involving suffering, like cancer, it's difficult for us to imagine any good outcomes. Yet the Bible assures us that "all the promises of God are 'Yes' in Christ" (2 Corinthians 1:20).

My cancer diagnosis and subsequent journey put God's promises to the test. The results were indisputable. God used everything, and I mean everything, for my good and his glory. God used each appointment and procedure, the billing and the bandages, every experience related to my cancer, even the collateral damage. God used the people in my life, from my family and friends to doctors and strangers, and even my enemies. Jesus will let nothing be wasted (John 6:12b).

Being a pastor for almost twenty years has given me substantial and important experience with disease. I've walked with people and families through sickness, including cancer, and all kinds of challenges; some unimaginable. I've been a shepherd in the valley of the shadow of death. I've learned from the people I've cared for and been inspired by them.

Being a pastor has also taught me a lot about God. I am fortunate to have received my seminary education from one of the best schools in the world. More importantly, I've experienced God. I know God's heart of compassion, God's promises and desires, God's strength to save, and all God can do in our lives. I know the word of God as "a lamp for my feet, a light on my path" (Psalm 119:105). Most importantly, I know Jesus, the healing balm of Gilead (Jeremiah 8:22). I can see him now carrying the one lost sheep on his shoulders back into the fold. I can hear

Jesus asking, "Do you want to be made well?" And I know that he is able! I have preached and taught it all for a long time, and I've experienced it in my own life.

In reflecting on my cancer experience, I could see how my lifelong Christian faith, my connection with the church, and especially my many years as a pastor had been so helpful. The disease demanded everything I had and more. Writing also made me increasingly aware of and concerned for those who might not have these kinds of resources available to them. In this book, I've attempted to share with others what helped me, along with the challenges, blessings, and experiences. I hope I can be helpful to others.

I never envisioned this being a book about how I was cured of cancer. I believed God would physically heal me, but I felt called to write a book about the space between diagnosis and a cure. I wanted to explore the other kinds of healing God can do in us in that time. I wrote most of this book while I waited, hoped for, and continued to believe God would heal me physically. Everything written here is based on my real-time journal entries as I lived from diagnosis through each subsequent day until my first cancer-free scan almost two years later. I wrote while knowing full well the abysmal survival rate for my disease. I wrote in that space for almost two years. I wrote knowing cancer would still be part of my life even when it was "gone." The medications and scans would continue.

What's unique about my story is that I write about all kinds of amazing healing—relational, emotional, spiritual, and more happening in my life while I still had cancer. Not when I had finally tidied up my life, but when a hurricane had made a mess of everything. I share how God worked in the chaos of cancer to make me whole. It's real.

I believe this book can provide a helpful and hopeful vision for approaching and living with cancer. A vision is a picture of our desired future. A vision has the power to give us direction and keep us moving forward. Once we have a vision, we can pursue it with all our might. Knowing where you're going makes all the difference. The Bible says, "Where there is no vision, the people perish" (Proverbs 29:18, KJV).

A cancer diagnosis shatters your vision and makes it hard to even plan your next step. A single-minded determination on "beating cancer," "winning the battle," or "being a survivor" can be counterproductive, insufficient, and limiting. Yes, we should pray for physical healing. But we can and should also pray for God to use our cancer experience to heal all our brokenness. Whether physical healing comes relatively soon, after a long journey, or doesn't come at all, God can accomplish immense good in our lives. So often, the most difficult times are the most transformative. I hope this book helps the reader envision the wide and spectacular array of personal healing God can accomplish in our lives. Some things are more important than physical healing.

Cancer patients need a vision that is bigger than physical healing. At some point, many cancer patients discern and come to peace with the realization that God's healing will come through death and entrance into the heavenly kingdom, where there is no more death, pain, or sickness. Hopefully, you will be physically healed. God may promise you that. But if not, all is not lost. All can still be gained. Envision your life, however long that may be, as a time for a more complete healing of your mind, soul, spirit, and relationships. Dream about what else God might do in this time. Mend a relationship. Reconnect or deepen your relationship with God. Enable you to provide a faithful witness. Physical healing is just a small part of the saving work of Jesus Christ.

In my book, I share fifteen facets of healing I experienced in the first two years of my cancer journey. Each chapter reflects on one of those areas of healing. Together they form a stunning, diamond-like array of what God can do—even in disease. The first chapter addresses courage. While cancer scared me and my fears surrounded me, God used cancer to make me more courageous. I share those lessons. I write about one of the most courageous people I have ever known and the inspiring way she lived with cancer for several years. And I share some of the ways I saw myself being braver, and the difference that made in my cancer experience. The following chapters follow the same format

Even though the "Healing" chapter ends with my cancer-free scan, everything up to that point is written from the perspective of someone still waiting for that wonderful news. This book remains, from start to finish, a book about how God can use cancer to cure you, wherever you are in your cancer experience. Even after a cancer-free scan, God will continue to use the disease for our good and his glory.

Lest it sound like I'm giving kudos to cancer, let me be clear—I am not. Cancer is a terrible disease. It's painful, scary, hard, heart-breaking, and it takes loved ones away. The mortal threat, the sickening drugs, the surgeries, the costliness, the uncertainly and worry that it will return—it's all horrible. Unanswered prayers for physical healing add to the pain. The fact that some readers are still grieving and missing loved ones lost to cancer challenges my message that anything good could possibly come from it. I am by no means telling you everything is going to be great and easy because you have cancer.

As Christians, we believe "*all things* work together for good for those who love God" (Romans 8:28). God can take and use what is bad for our good. That includes cancer. God takes death and turns it into a resurrection life. Nothing is impossible for God! When we give our lives to Christ, he and his resurrection power live in us! We are refined and tested in the furnace of affliction (Isaiah 48:10). We glory in our sufferings (Romans 5:3).

This book isn't a collection of sermons, a theological dissertation, or a subversive attempt to change your worldview. I promise. It's my story. I invite you to hear it, find yourself in it, and enjoy it. If it opens you up to the possibility of believing in God, helps you catch a glimpse of God in your situation, or more importantly, leads you to faith in Jesus Christ and a relationship with him, I will be ecstatic. I will also be very happy if my story gives you any amount of joy, encouragement, and hope.

This book is written, first and foremost, for cancer patients, their spouses and children, family and friends, and other loved ones. It's written for those shocked by a cancer diagnosis. I believe my experience and approach will be helpful to someone recently diagnosed, as well as those surviving year after year. It's for fellow sojourners looking for mile markers, support, and blessings on the cancer journey.

Cancer is not the world's only antagonist. It is not the only disease. Your disease may be another health crisis. Your disease may be a broken marriage, extended unemployment, financial brokenness, unresolved anger, or something else. Whatever it is, I hope this book will give you hope. God can mend what's been broken. God can heal it, and God can use it to heal you.

"For nothing will be impossible with God"
—Luke 1:37, ESV

Courage

I'm not sure how long I had been coughing, but it had been long enough. The pain in my side felt like broken ribs whenever I coughed. Sleeping on my side had become impossible. The over-the-counter pain medication and cough drops weren't helping enough. I could feel my voice weakening more quickly, which isn't good for a preacher.

My wife, Amy, had been concerned for a while and suggested I see my doctor. When she started hearing similar coughs on the pulmonary floor of the hospital, where she was working as a requirement of nursing school, she insisted I go.

I went to see my general physician. He suggested that allergies might be to blame and prescribed some medication. Just to be safe, he sent me to have an X-ray of my lungs.

A few hours later, my doctor called and told me I had a golf-ball-sized mass in my right lung. I needed some more scans, an appointment with a pulmonary specialist, and possibly another with an oncologist.

A few days and a couple of scans later, Amy and I met with the pulmonologist. Scrolling and clicking through the digital images, he showed us the golf-ball-sized mass in my right lung, and several other places of concern—my sternum, spine, kidney, and neck.

His diagnosis didn't take long. He straightened his back, turned towards us, and told us what we didn't want to hear:

"It's lung cancer. Stage four. Quite advanced. A classic case."

After a few moments, Amy broke the awkward silence. "But he's not a smoker. He's never smoked. How can this happen?"

Equally stunned, I added, "I'm not around second-hand smoke. My parents didn't smoke. There's no family history of cancer. I'm in perfect health. I feel good. I'm only forty-five years old."

"He exercises regularly, " Amy said. "He ran five miles yesterday."

The doc said something about how many people in the U.S. are diagnosed with lung cancer each year, and how many of those are non-smokers. He talked about some of the encouraging treatment options. He spoke about the biopsy I would need ASAP, something called a bronchoscopy. It was all a blur.

Having run out of questions, Amy and I sat in disbelief.

Breaking the silence, with both matter-of-factness and compassion, he added, "It's just bad luck."

After a slow and silent walk back to the parking deck, I pulled out into a torrential rain pour. My windshield wipers couldn't go fast enough, and the traffic couldn't move slower. A long line of red brake lights lit up the main corridor through campus. Red lights flashed off occasionally as if we were going to move.

While sitting in the car, I had never felt so afraid. The bottom had just fallen out of my life—stage four lung cancer. I tried to push back the fear. I gripped the steering wheel as I recited a few Bible verses. "Do not fear, for I am with you; do not be dismayed, for I am your God. I will strengthen you and help you" (Isaiah 41:10). "Take courage! It is I. Don't be afraid" (Mathew 14:27). "Perfect love casts out fear" (1 John 4:18, ESV).

I called Amy as I waited behind the red lights. We had driven separate vehicles. We weren't ready to go home and tell our kids the news. We needed time to gather ourselves and figure out what to say.

We decided to stop by for a short visit with Roger and Jean, members of our church. We had met them about a year earlier when we moved to the area so I could serve as senior pastor of the United Methodist Church, where they were members. They were among the first people to reach out to us. Their genuine interest amazed us. Over the past year, they had become like family to us.

Jean led the weekly women's prayer group and the Wednesday intercessory prayer group, two positions she had held for forty years. She seemed like a saint and my favorite elementary school teacher combined. Roger, a renowned yet unassuming professor of electro-bioengineering at the nearby university, slipped inconspicuously in and out of Sunday worship weekly. Both attended every week unless they were out of town visiting their beloved grandchildren. Roger and Jean put the grand in grandparent.

Both were among the most generous, gentle, kind, supportive, wise, discerning, and calm people we had ever known. We could count on them to listen, understand, and give us encouragement and good advice. They were exactly what we needed, and they lived between the hospital and our home.

Jean welcomed us. After hugging Amy and me, Jean handed me a small, thick white envelope. Without much thought, although curious, I put it in my coat pocket and took a seat on the sofa across from Roger. Amy and I told them all about the doctor's report, the next steps, our feelings, and our fears, especially about telling our kids. Jean prayed for us. Amy and I held hands. I can't remember Jean's words, but I'll never forget the comfort of her praying for us. After a few more minutes of receiving their wonderful encouragement and support, we said our goodbyes and headed home.

At home, I took off my jacket. As I hung it in the hall closet, I remembered the envelope Jean had given me and pulled it out. I felt the thickness of the postcard-sized white envelope and imagined it might contain a few bills of cash. *We'll need it.* I turned it over and read the words written on the envelope: "Fear Chasers."

I decided to go up to our bedroom and open the envelope in private before talking with our kids. I needed a moment to collect myself.

I sat on the chair beside my bed. Interested and feeling grateful for Jean, I opened the envelope and removed a small piece of yellow notebook paper from it. On the first lines, Jean had written, "The Bible, with its realistic knowledge of the human heart, repeats three hundred and sixty-five times the words fear not." She footnoted her source below and signed her name at the bottom of the page.

Inside the envelope, Jean had placed about a dozen white index cards. I removed them all and shuffled through them. All appeared to be structured the same. I slid one out of the deck for a more careful look and set the others on the table. I took note of Jean's excellent penmanship and the neatly handwritten cursive. On one side of the card, in the center, Jean had written, "Fear Chaser." On the other side, she had written a short Bible verse. I took a deep breath, centered myself, and read the verse.

"Be strong and courageous. Do not be afraid or terrified because of them, for the LORD your God goes with you; he will never leave you nor forsake you" (Deuteronomy 31:6).

As I read the words slowly, repeating them, I felt God's strength and courage filling my heart. I again felt the comfort of Jean's prayer for us. In some way, I felt the fears being chased away.

I joined Amy downstairs, and we gathered the kids in the living room. I could tell they were trying to be strong when I told them about the doctor's visit, the report, my cancer, and what would happen next. Amy helped fill in the details. We listened to their concerns and answered their questions as best we could. I assured them God would be with us, help us, and provide everything we need. They didn't need to be afraid. After that, I said a short prayer for our family.

Despite putting on a brave face for our kids, I was still scared. In my entire life, I had never been so afraid.

A simple internet search found a barrage of frightening facts. Lung cancer is the scariest cancer of them all. Lung cancer takes more lives than breast cancer, colon cancer, and prostate cancer combined. It's the number one cancer killer. I read about the high mortality rates, the low percentage of five-year survivorship, and the shockingly small amount of money spent annually on lung cancer research.[1] All of this scared me.

I didn't fear death. I had faith in Jesus, and I believed I would go to heaven when I died. My fear was that death would come too soon. I had what my kids call *FOMO*, the fear of missing out. I feared I would miss out on my children's graduations, weddings, and all the other special moments. I feared I would miss out on spending the rest of my life with Amy. The best for us was yet to come.

With the diagnosis of cancer and each following step, I encountered new fears. It's like the creepy cancer bus pulled up to my front door, and all kinds of fears unloaded into my life. The fear of death and FOMO were just the beginning. After that, came *scanxiety*, the fear of the scan results. *What are they going to find?* And the fear that the cancer has suddenly spread everywhere. *It could be in my liver, spine, brain...* Then came the fear of biopsies, results, and treatments. *Can my type of cancer be treated effectively? Is there medication? What kind? Will I need radiation? Surgery?* There was the fear of insurance companies. *Will my required treatment and medication be approved?* I feared not being able to get the drugs I needed more than the side effects. I feared the hospital billing departments and running out of money. I feared how disruptive cancer would be to my life and my family. *How will this impact my kids' schoolwork?* I feared I would lose my job. *Will the church want a pastor with cancer?* The fears kept coming.

Honestly, I struggled with a lot of fears before cancer. We'll call them my pre-existing fears: the fear of failure, the fear of not being good enough, the fear of being rejected, the fear of criticism, the fear of asking for help. I felt ill-equipped to deal with a whole new busload of fears.

Each year, our family enjoys watching *A Charlie Brown Christmas*. In one scene of the movie, Lucy attempts to diagnose what's wrong with Charlie Brown. She hypothesizes that he might have a phobia and runs through a long list of possibilities, including the fear of responsibility and the fear of cats. She names and defines them all, but none seem to be Charlie's issue.

Exasperated, Lucy says, "Do you think you have pantophobia?"

"What's pantophobia?" Charlie replies.

"The fear of everything."

"That's it!" Charlie says.[2]

Between my old fears and my new cancer fears, I was starting to feel like Charlie, afraid of everything. I felt like I was drowning in my fears; they were getting the best of me. Good grief!

In the months following, I took a Fear Chaser to each CAT scan and every appointment. I may have looked silly, but I didn't care. Each Wednesday, Jean brought me a new Fear Chaser, sliding it under my office door or placing it on my desk. She did this for nearly a year and a half. I have kept them all clasped together and sitting on my desk, where they are always handy and helpful. Every time, the words did their job—reassuring me of God's presence and love, and *casting out fear* (1 John 4:18, ESV).

At one of my first appointments, I waited anxiously for seventy-five minutes in a crowded hospital waiting room to see my doctor. Finally, my pager activated. Its vibrations and flashing red lights startled me. Alas, my time had come. I rushed to the doors where the nurses met each patient to take them back to the observation room.

A minute or two passed, and still, no one had come to meet me. The doors remained shut. Meanwhile, the pager continued to vibrate and flash in my hand. I looked over to the receptionist, now busy attending to another patient. With a nod, she assured me I was in the right place.

Suddenly, I felt alone. It was like a scene from a sci-fi horror movie where everyone disappears, and you are left alone in an empty place. Everyone in the clinic disappeared. I had never felt so forsaken. The pager in my hand vibrated and flashed like a time bomb soon to explode. *No one is coming. This is the end. My life is over!* Sheer terror seized me.

After what felt like an eternity, I heard my name being called from far away. I looked around, saw the crowded waiting room, and spotted my nurse standing in front of a different door at the other end of the clinic, about twenty-five feet away. I went to her, and without a word, she took the pager from me and led me into the clinic.

In my devotional time the next morning, I reflected on how afraid and alone I had felt, and then read again the words from my first Fear Chaser: "Be strong and courageous. Do not be afraid or terrified because of them, for the LORD your God goes with you; he will never leave you nor forsake you" (Deuteronomy 31:6).

God seemed to be speaking to me. *"You weren't alone yesterday. You will never be alone. I am always with you. You have nothing to fear."*

I regretted having allowed myself to become so afraid. I could have felt strong and courageous as I waited in the clinic. I was not alone. I had my wife with me, my parents, and tons of support. I had a pocket full of Fear Chasers. Most importantly, God was with me and always would be through every step of this cancer journey.

I recalled Jesus' promise, "Be sure of this: I am with you always, even to the end of the age" (Matthew 28:20b, NLT).

The Bible is clear. God doesn't want us to be afraid. I knew that, but it was hard not to be. I needed to be reminded. Knowing my heart and needs, God often led me to Bible verses and stories about overcoming fear.

"So do not fear, for I am with you; do not be dismayed, for I am your God. I will strengthen you and help you; I will uphold you with my righteous right hand" (Isaiah 41:10).

I recalled Jesus' promise to his disciples. As a minister, I had offered these words of comfort to many.

"Peace I leave with you; my peace I give you. I do not give to you as the world gives. Do not let your hearts be troubled and do not be afraid" (John 14:27).

The Bible assures us, "There is no fear in love, but perfect love casts out fear. For fear has to do with punishment" (1 John 4:18a, ESV).

Jesus' death on the cross and his resurrection had saved me from death. He had cast out my fear of death. I also had the assurance of Jesus' love and presence with me every day. I knew he would faithfully shepherd me through my cancer journey.

God also brought to my mind many examples of courageous people found in the Bible. I thought of Caleb calling his fellow Israelites to be brave as they prepared to take their Promised Land from enemies so big that they made everyone else feel like hopeless grasshoppers. "We should go up and take possession of the land, for we can certainly do it" (Numbers 13:30).

I thought of the woman in Mark who had suffered from chronic bleeding for many years. She pushed through her fear to touch Jesus' cloak because she believed he could heal her, and he did (Mark 5:25-34). I thought of Peter, whose name means *rock*, and him climbing out of the boat and walking on the stormy water, toward Jesus (Matthew 14:29, NIV).

Early on, I thought of one of the most courageous people I had ever known who had faced cancer—my mother-in-law, Dot. When I entered her life, after I had captured her daughter's heart, Dot was in the third year of her five-year battle with a rare and aggressive type of ovarian cancer. By the time I met her, she had endured multiple surgeries, powerful and debilitating chemotherapy and radiation, every imaginable scan and test possible, and appointments with specialists across the country. Doctors didn't expect her to live many months longer.

I wouldn't have known it, though. Dot was fun, joyful, loving, and determined. She wore her wigs well and always put on makeup. "It's better to look good than to feel good," she would always say. The only thing that gave her cancer away was the little bucket she always kept at her side because of nausea caused by the chemotherapy continually being pumped into her body through a permanent IV.

Her children called her "the killer" in honor of her tenacity. When the hospital would call trying to collect on the $100,000 balance on her account, she'd shout across the room to Bob, my father-in-law, "Pay them a dollar, Bob!" She was not afraid of the insurance company or anyone else.

As a final attack against her cancer, Dot endured the most invasive and risky surgery, a sixteen-hour-long, life-risking procedure. I shudder as I recall the doctors describing to the family their plans for the surgery, especially the "shake and bake" part. They would open her abdomen and pour chemotherapy medication directly onto the tumors and swish it around them. The tumors were like Velcro, clinging to her organs. The surgeons planned to cut away as much as possible and then hoped the chemo would kill or control the rest. It was risky, but it was the only way.

As we sat and listened, scared out of our minds, Dot showed no fear. She nodded, confirmed her understanding, and signed the required paperwork. When the doctors left, she asked Amy for her purse and pulled from it her makeup. "Well, my Darlings, it's better to look good than to feel good."

I marveled at her courage. We all did.

Miraculously, Dot made it home alive. After a long recovery, although plagued with chronic nausea, tethered to her pail, and unsure how much time she had left, she continued to live courageously. She fought to live long enough to meet, hold, and kiss her first grandchild, Marcie. She came to visit us as often as she could, and treasured every moment.

We engaged in many deep spiritual conversations. Dot was a faithful Christian. She had been through a lot in her life, including the death of her oldest child, Marcie, our daughter's namesake, in a car accident at age sixteen. Somehow Dot had held on to her faith and held her family together. It wasn't easy. She drew her strength and courage from the Lord. I admired her faith.

We talked a lot about me feeling called to leave my job, go to seminary, and become a pastor. Since I had met Dot, the call had become stronger. I was afraid to do it, but Dot persistently encouraged me to go for it. To help me overcome my fears, I think she made me her family's pastor. I became the one called upon to pray at all family gatherings and to pray with her privately after she had become bedridden.

When we knew the end of her life was close at hand, she asked me to gather the family together in the family room and lead a time of prayer and encourage them. Later that evening, Dot shoed everyone else away until it was just the two of us. I held her hand and prayed softly for Dot. She was at peace and not afraid, courageous to the end. Moments later, I felt the presence of God come, and she died holding my hand. She was fifty-nine.

Unbeknownst to me, Dot had requested that I preach at her funeral and give her eulogy. As my father in law, Bob, began to make plans for the funeral with their church, he asked me to fulfill this great honor. Of course, I did, and as God and Dot would have it, this would be my first sermon ever preached. After that day, I answered God's call. A few months later, I left my job, started seminary, and was appointed pastor of my first church.

Dot's courageous witness continued to inspire me. Now her brave spirit encouraged me to face my own cancer courageously. I hoped I could be half "the killer" Dot was and give my family and others the same powerful witness.

I wanted to say goodbye to other long-held fears of mine. For so long, I had been afraid of not being good enough, not being liked, and being unwanted. These and other fears had held me back in my pastoral leadership. On so many occasions, I hadn't spoken the truth about important issues facing the church. My fear of failure had kept me from taking risks that could have been very rewarding to me and others. Fear of disappointing my kids had kept me from making important parenting decisions.

I longed for God to use my cancer experience, with all its fearsomeness, to make me more courageous. Already, each scary situation had been an opportunity to choose courage over fear—telling my kids I had cancer, talking with the hospital's billing department, reading the insurance company's paperwork, learning more about my disease, having my first ever scans, having blood drawn. Each time I exercised my courage, my courage grew a little more.

The days following my meeting with the pulmonologist were frantic and frightening—more scans and tests, calls and appointments, and a referral to an oncologist.

In the middle of this immense uncertainty and overwhelming fear, I picked up my Bible for my morning devotions and turned to John's gospel. My daily reading was the story of Jesus raising Lazarus from the dead.

It's a great story. Lazarus and his sisters, Martha and Mary, are close friends of Jesus. Lazarus gets sick and is at death's door. The sisters call for Jesus to come home. Jesus inexplicably waits two more days, until after Lazarus has died, to come. Jesus arrives and tells Martha not to worry. "I am the resurrection and the life. The one who believes in me will live, even though they die; and whoever lives by believing in me will never die" (John 11:25-26). After proclaiming those words, he calls Lazarus out of the tomb, bringing him back to life.

As I read the story, one sentence stopped me in my tracks: "This sickness will not end in death. No, it is for God's glory so that God's Son may be glorified through it" (John 11:4).

I could hear Jesus speaking those words to me. *David, this sickness will not end in death.* I felt his presence in the room.

I heard the promise of my share in the resurrection, eternal life, and heaven. But I heard Jesus say something more. I heard him say, *I'm going to heal you physically,* and *I'm going to use you and this sickness to bring glory to my name.*

I struggled to wrap my head around what Jesus had said. I was certain I had heard him correctly. I considered for a moment that Jesus might have meant that something else would kill me other than cancer, but that didn't sound very Christ-like. I thought about people I knew and loved who hadn't been healed. But still, I believed Jesus. My cancer would not end in death.

With those words from Jesus, the earth shook, and my existential fears were put on notice. If you no longer need to fear death, what else could you possibly need to fear?

Grace

I dreaded telling my church I had cancer. I worried that they wouldn't want a sick pastor who required their care. After all, my job as a pastor was to care for them. I worried that they would not want a pastor who couldn't give 100 percent.

I had been their pastor just a little more than one year, and everything was going great. I didn't want my health to jeopardize that.

Once the doctors confirmed the golf-ball-sized mass in my lung was cancer, I had to let the congregation know. Amy and I had told our family and close friends, and I feared word might get out. I decided to send a message out via email Saturday night, and make an announcement Sunday in worship. I painstakingly crafted that message.

> Doctors recently found a golf-ball-sized tumor in my lung. Testing has confirmed that it's lung cancer, stage four. I'm working with doctors to determine my course of treatment. I am encouraged and trust God to heal me. Thank you in advance for your love and support. I feel great and will continue working and giving my ministry 100 percent.

Never had I been so afraid to send an email. I copied everyone I thought needed to be among those first in the know—my supervisors, mentors, and close colleagues. I took a deep breath, pressed send, turned the computer off, and went to bed.

In the morning, with some trepidation, I checked my messages. Emails and text messaged had started pouring in right after I had sent my message. All night long and into the morning, members of the congregation had emailed with promises of prayer, words of encouragement, pledges of support, offers to help, and affirmations of love and concern. The intercessory prayer team had been activated. A meal train had been started. The knitting team had prayer blankets ready for each member of my family. Key leaders and staff had pledged their support. There were countless offers to help.

In worship, I read my emailed message to the congregation before I preached. Their faces showed heartbreak for me, and the love, compassion, faith, and readiness to help that I had read in their messages to me.

At the conclusion of worship, I stood in front of the congregation to give the benediction. As I began to speak, Rick, a lay leader of the congregation, hurried to the front and gently took the microphone from me. He asked my family—Amy, Marcie, Hannah, and Caleb—to stand with me. Looking at the congregation and us, he pledged the congregation's love and support, *no matter what*. He then invited everyone to come circle around me and lay hands on me as he led a prayer for us. In an instant, the entire congregation, two hundred people or more, engulfed us in a tight embrace. In the middle, I wrapped my arms around my kids and Amy. Rick prayed, and I felt unbelievably reassured of the congregation's love for us.

That same Sunday, in our next worship service, I again announced my cancer update. As I spoke, surveying the faces of all the attendees, my gaze locked in on Pastor Harvin's. He was seated at the back-left corner. He leaned forward and sat up straight, listening attentively. In that moment, I heard God say to me; *Pastor Harvin can be helpful to you.*

Pastor Harvin, a retired United Methodist pastor, had recently started attending our church. We had worked together a few times over the years. He had retired as senior pastor of one of the largest churches in our conference. I remembered him being a great preacher, a natural with people, kind, and funny.

A couple of days later, Pastor Harvin invited me to meet him for coffee. In the café, we sat at a corner table, and he cut to the chase.

"While I was in worship Sunday and you were making your announcement, I heard the Lord calling me to help you."

As I sat in awe of the divine providence of God, David shared how, with each passing hour, the urgency to see me had become unbearable.

"So, " he concluded, "here I am, at your service."

Pastor Harvin offered to cover all my ministry responsibilities as needed, preach weekly, visit the sick, even attend all the committee meetings. And, he continued, "God forbid, if you need to take a few weeks or a few months off, maybe take some medical leave, I would be willing to fill in as an interim, for free."

I knew he could do my job, all of it, surely better than I could. Still, I felt a wave of anxiety roll over me. I wasn't thinking about taking any time off from work. I didn't even want to put the idea on the table. I was so thrown off by the phrases "leave of absence" and "medical leave" that I almost missed the miracle. It felt reminiscent of the angel of God, calling Peter and Cornelius to meet (Acts 10:1-11:18, ESV). I could barely comprehend Pastor's Harvin's gracious and amazing offer.

As much as I appreciated Pastor Harvin's offer, the idea of taking a leave of absence horrified me. Would the church want me when I got back? Would my family be provided for? More importantly, what would I do with my life? Who would I be if I couldn't work? What worth would I have? My work meant everything to me.

My dad instilled into me the value of hard work. He left early each morning, worked long days, and gained great success as an executive. When he got home, he changed clothes and got to work on projects around the house and the nearly fourteen acres of property. Building, renovating, repairing, or remodeling. It never stopped. My dad's skills continued to amaze me, even as an adult. He taught us that if you work hard enough, you can accomplish anything. Nothing beats the satisfaction of a job well done.

Dad kept my brothers and me busy at home. In addition to homework, we had our regular chores. Saturday mornings began with dad outside our bedroom windows, revving up his high-powered weed eater and shouting, between the engine's blasts, "Rise and shine!" We spent the day working, mowing, bush hogging, weed eating, trimming, raking, cleaning the pool, and whatever else needed to be done. Dad was always working, and our working hard at his side pleased him.

I worked from the time I was old enough to get a job—flipping burgers, bagging groceries, and even telemarketing. I worked some while I was in college, mostly for spending-money. When I graduated from college, I got a job right away. I quickly discovered cold calling wasn't my calling, left my sales job, and went to work at a small print shop as a graphic designer. I enjoyed that even though the pay and hours were terrible. The place reeked of cigarettes, but I enjoyed the work and met Amy there, in a cloud of smoke. After that, I worked for my dad for five years at Quality Truck Bodies and Repair, Inc., a business he had just bought and started operating. I worked alongside him, learning even more about hard work until my call to ministry sent me off to work for the Lord.

Over the next twenty years, I pastored four churches. I worked hard at preaching, striving weekly to bring an engaging message. I loved, cared, and prayed for my parishioners. I worked hard to support and empower staff, leaders, and committees. I cast vision, set goals, tracked progress. I gave my all to stewardship campaigns, fundraising efforts, crisis, and conflict management. Consequently, I had moved up in the ranks over the years, until most recently being appointed to serve my largest congregation yet, with a talented multiple-person staff.

The work of ministry meant everything to me. Living into my calling gave my life purpose and meaning. I felt a sense of accomplishment. Seeing the difference it made in peoples' lives provided affirmation. Dealing effectively with challenges gave me great satisfaction. Work drove me and energized me. It allowed me to provide for my family in a way that made me feel good. It blessed me with opportunities to move up if I kept working hard.

Cancer threatened to take away my ability to work. I feared that if I took *any* time off, the church might think I needed to take even more. The more time off I took, the more likely I'd lose my job. So I doubled down in the face of cancer. Through the appointments, continued coughing, my aching side, and the waiting and uncertainty, and everything else, I worked extra hard. I refused to take off even a day or two. I convinced myself that doing so was unnecessary. I thanked Pastor Harvin for his offer but told him and others that the best thing I could do for myself and my family was to continue working.

As I did so, determined not to allow cancer to cost me my job, I found myself working harder than ever. Somehow, during my mad dash, the absurdity of it all came into sharp focus—I was more afraid of losing my job than I was of losing my life to cancer.

Over the years, I had talked with my counselor, my best friends, and Amy about my struggle with workaholism. Amy had expressed her frustration many times, but how do you argue with a man working for God? I understood it was wrong, and promised to do better. Truthfully, being a workaholic, was like a badge of honor to me.

Now, as I pondered the possibility of losing my job, I could see for the first time the severity of my workaholism and its damaging effects. I was grossly dependent on work to give me purpose, love, and security. I needed work like an alcoholic needs liquor. I could see the damage it had caused to my family and me.

With that dependency on work came ridiculous pressure to always prove myself, work harder than anyone else, take no time off, make no mistakes, and avoid criticism at all costs. In turn, I gave so much of myself to work that I had little or nothing left for my marriage, children, family, or friends. I wouldn't even take care of myself.

In all my fretting about work, I began to think more about grace. I knew that's what I needed. Our tendency as humans is to depend on our works to fix everything, from the smallest problem to our relationship with God. The Bible tells us to rely on the grace of God. God has done all the needed work for us.

"For it is by grace you have been saved, through faith—and this is not from yourselves, it is the gift of God—not by works, so that no one can boast" (Ephesians 2:8-9).

For over twenty years, I had preached grace. From the start, I loved the United Methodist Church's emphasis on grace. That's why I became a pastor. We named our firstborn child Marcie Grace. I taught classes on grace. I preached countless sermons on the topic. "Grace Anatomy," a five-part sermon series, remains one of my all-time favorites. A year before my cancer diagnosis, I had been appointed to lead a church with a vision to be a community of faith "living in grace."

I like the United Methodist's definition of grace. "By grace, we mean the undeserved, unmerited, and loving action of God in human existence through the ever-present Holy Spirit."[3] I think grace can be distilled to the *undeserved love of God (ULOG)*. I taught my congregation ULOG to help them remember. I needed to remember, too.

Grace is all about God's loving action. Because God loves us, God acts. God's love isn't just talk. God's love activated the creation of the world and everything in it. God created us to love us and for us to love God. When God saw the world in need of saving, he took loving action. For God so loved the world he *gave* his only son Jesus (John 3:16). In love, God acts to provide all that we need—physically, spiritually, emotionally—every day. God gives us our daily bread. God raises us from the dead and gives us eternal life. Every good and perfect gift comes from God. God's loving action is not just in someone else's life or some other world; it's in my human existence. It's not limited to certain places or times; God loves us through his ever-present Holy Spirit.

What makes God's love grace is that it's undeserved. We haven't done anything to earn it. The Bible bluntly tells us, "...all have sinned and fallen short of the glory of God" (Romans 3:23). We have failed God, worked against God's purposes and ignored God. Everyone's sins are equally grievous in the face of God. We all deserve death and punishment. God loves us anyway, every one of us, not just the loveable. God gave his one and only perfect Son to save scallywag sinners. Having given his Son, God goes on to give us everything else, all the riches of heaven.

When you have an awareness of God's love and an awareness of your undeserved-ness, you can start living in grace. Jesus is all about grace. He is the literal embodiment of God's grace. When the church lives up to its full potential, it's a community of people living in grace.

For me to live in grace, I had to stop trying to earn, deserve, and work for everything. I had to trust God to continue loving and providing for me no matter what, even though I didn't deserve it. I also needed to have greater faith in the church. I had to trust that the followers of Jesus Christ would love me no matter what. I could slow down and take time for my family and for myself. I could let the church love, care, and support me. Their love wasn't something I had to earn or deserve. It was grace!

Living in grace challenged my faith. I had to believe in God's unconditional love for me. God would love me just as much, whether sick or healthy, able, or disabled. I had to believe I am good and worthy even if I can't work as much or at all, and even if I need others to help me. I had to believe my family and other people would love me unconditionally.

I began to feel in my struggle to live in grace that God would use my cancer to cure me of my workaholism. God would show me how to live not by work, but by grace.

A couple of days after my cancer announcement, Helen stopped by the office to ask if she could set up a "meal train" for our family. It would save us time, energy, and money, and give the congregation opportunities to show their love and support. Helen passionately led and served our church's food ministry. After inquiring with Amy as to preferable days and times for meal delivery, dietary requirements, and favorite types of foods, she quickly got to work. Within a couple of hours, she had a schedule set to bring dinner three times a week, and an unprecedented number of congregants on board to make it happen. With that, the meal train started rolling. *Chew! Chew!*

That evening, the meal train made its first stop. Robert and Sharon brought several frozen meals, home-grown vegetables, and completely astonished us with the gift of a brand-new, full-sized storage freezer. As Sharon told Amy about tonight's meal, Robert unloaded the freezer from his truck, rolled it into place in the garage, plugged it in, and stacked several meals inside it. Every day since the freezer has stood as a powerful reminder of the congregation's unconditional love for me. It's a freezer full of grace.

Two days later, the doorbell rang, and I opened the door and found Sarah standing on the step, with several plastic grocery bags hanging from both forearms, and she was holding a few more in her hands. With a big, bright smile, she said, "Hey Giras, are you ready for a fiesta!"

We watched in awe as Sarah began emptying the contents of her bags onto the kitchen counter: two Mexican casseroles—essentially, two giant enchiladas—two bags of tortilla chips, a jar of their family's favorite salsa, a bowl of guacamole, a casserole dish filled with Mexican rice, a tossed salad, salad dressings, desert, and bottles of Mexican sodas—orange, cherry, lime, and more. *Loco!*

As she set up our fiesta, she encouraged Amy and our children, listening carefully to each, all the while smiling and laughing. The many overflowing bags seemed to be filled with her love for us.

Sarah asked me to retrieve one last bag from her car. On the street, I popped open the hatchback, looked in, and spotted the bag. Inside of it, I found a six-pack of Mexican beer with a small plastic bag filled with pre-cut limes stuffed between the bottle necks. I looked around, both amused and amazed by Sarah's love, and would not have been at all surprised to find a sombrero and a piñata.

Day after day, one amazing meal after another showed up on our doorstep. We were amazed at the thoughtful preparation and grateful for each dish. A few meals went above and beyond anything, we would have ever expected.

Josephine and Carrol hired a caterer to cook and deliver multiple full-sized serving trays filled with southern fried chicken, homemade macaroni and cheese, country beans, and banana pudding. It looked like we were having a family reunion.

Barry brought a big beautiful beef brisket simmering in a rich aromatic sauce, along with pieces of carrots, potatoes, and onion. He had cooked the brisket "low and slow" for the past twelve hours.

Kim delivered her four-course meal on a wooden tray that looked like something we would have received at a bed and breakfast. She even placed a small vase with a few fresh cut flowers on the corner.

I will always remember one of the simpler meals. After a Sunday worship service, Fred, a senior statesman of the church, stopped by my office and handed me two small, worn, plastic containers and a small baggie containing a dinner roll. Lovingly, he said to me, "Nancy and I don't cook much, but we wanted to give you something to show our love for you and your family."

A half-hour later, I arrived home to find the rest of the family had gone out to lunch without me. Left to fend for myself, I opened Fred's containers, grabbed a fork and a plate, and enjoyed a modest portion of the tasty green bean casserole, a dinner roll, and a serving of delicious fig pudding.

For more than six months, the grace train delivered meals. Eventually, my kids started asking when we could cook again. When I thought we might not need it anymore, I tried to stop the train, but the congregation kept signing up. On one occasion, Kim shared with me how excited she was to hear that another member who had signed up to bring us dinner had gotten sick and could no longer bring a meal as planned. The member's sickness had opened a slot on the schedule and gave Kim, to her enormous and scrumptious delight, another opportunity to cook for us.

The meal train helped more than we could have imagined. We always had a delicious and nutritious meal, usually with a desert. We never had to think about food or run to the grocery store. Each meal appeared like manna from heaven. We were able to focus on dealing with my cancer and getting well. The meal train was a tangible and tasty expression of what I needed most—grace.

Each meal expressed love for my family and me. People say the quickest way to a person's heart is through their stomach, and I knew each meal had been prepared and given in love. Each meal took time and energy. Some, like Kim, Barry, and Sarah, blew me away. So much love had been cooked into these meals. It was even better than having your mom bring you homemade chicken noodle soup when you're sick.

Talk about amazing grace! I had been the church's pastor for a little more than a year. I was still getting to know the congregation. Many meals came from people I didn't even know yet. I hadn't been their pastor long enough to do anything great as a leader. I had already made many mistakes. In my first year, I may have run off more sheep than I had brought into the flock. Despite all my "still giving it a 100 percent!" I had probably slowed down some and was not doing as much. I had not done anything to deserve these meals. I hadn't earned any of this. Nonetheless, the meals kept coming. Undeserved love—grace— kept coming.

The meals preached to the preacher. "Taste and see that the Lord is good" (Psalm 34:8). I would never have to earn or deserve God's love. God would always love me. The meals reassured me that the faithful members of my church would always love me, too. They would stand with me and support me no matter what. I didn't have to work for that either. I could rest secure in their undeserved love.

The church loved us in many other ways throughout those first few months of my cancer journey. Many people promised to pray for me and did so in a way I had never experienced—praying all night, all day, throughout the day, without ceasing, on their knees, in prayer groups, and at home.

One day, Maye came urgently to my office to tell me that she, too, had just been diagnosed with cancer. She said that every time she tried to pray for herself, she couldn't. The Lord led her to pray instead for me. While we were together, she wanted to pray for me and then have me pray for her.

I received cards daily. Sometimes they were shorts notes of encouragement. Other times they were longer prayers written to God on my behalf or testimonies of God's goodness in the sender's own cancer experience. They came from everywhere— every place I had ever lived, every church I had belonged to or served. I received cards from Africa. One of the most meaningful cards came from a man incarcerated in the local prison. He had heard about me through our prison ministry and wrote to encourage me, and enclosed a $100 gift card.

We received help with practical needs, cleaning our house, and doing our yardwork, giving our children rides to school, church, and activities. Many offered to drive me to my appointments, sit with me while I waited (now that's love), and take me home. A couple of folks offered their vacation homes so we could get away to the beach or the mountains whenever we wanted. Several people offered to help pay our medical bills. Amazing grace!

Looking back on all the ways the church gave me grace, undeserved love, the meal train stands out. I think of *The Ol' Graceliner* rolling down the track, delivering one grace-filled meal after another. *Chew! Chew!* Today, it's impossible for me to see a train or train track without thinking about my church's meal train and how it blessed my family and me.

In all the weeks since my cancer diagnosis, God had used my cancer to teach me about grace. Amazingly, the threat of not being able to work showed me more about God's unconditional love for me than anything else could have. The abundance of amazing grace had begun to set me free and cure my workaholism. I could stop pushing myself to work so hard. I didn't have to do everything. I was loved by God, by my family and friends, and by my church, no matter what. With their help, I could learn to live in grace.

Forgiveness

Immediately after my diagnosis of stage 4 lung cancer, messages of encouragement, love, and well-wishes poured in from every direction. People were praying for me all over the world. The outpouring of love humbled me, warmed my heart, and helped immensely.

However, among the hundreds of cards, emails, and text messages I received, a few were from people I did not want to hear from, people who had hurt me in different ways over the years.

A text message came from one of the leaders of a church I had previously served. He had hurt my family and me terribly. During my time there, I spent a lot of time with him and his wonderful family. I loved and admired him and enjoyed our work together. I had trusted him. When I found out he had been meeting with other leaders and members of our congregation behind my back and plotting to get rid of me, I was devastated. I had been lied to and betrayed, which deeply hurt. I made the painful decision to leave that church for another without knowing what the next church might be. Moving my family at that time was terrible for our kids, especially our oldest, a rising high school senior. It was such a painful move. I never wanted to hear from him or anyone else involved in that decision again.

His message didn't say much: "Praying for you and thinking about you." My eyes burned, and my heart palpitated when I read his name. I tightened my grip on the phone. Looking back, I'm surprised I didn't throw it against the wall. I deleted the message at the speed of light, like a kid whose mom had walked in on him while he was looking at something inappropriate on his phone. In an instant, it was gone, but the bad feelings remained.

Facebook and social media presented challenges. Among my several hundred virtual friends, there were several who had conspired in causing me harm at some point in my life. Their "likes" and encouraging comments and messages made my blood pressure surge. I unfriended them all.

As the loving messages poured in, almost all from people I loved and knew cared about me, I stood on alert, worrying what other unsolicited and unwanted messages I might receive. *I hope I don't hear from him. She had better not even think about contacting me!* In my absurdity, I realized that I felt anger and held resentment towards far too many people. A seemingly endless list of people had made me angry, let me down, or betrayed me. So many of the people who had once been part of my life, I had booted out and blacklisted.

All, in one way or another, had made me angry. I replayed in my head, the horrible things I had said or wanted to say. I remembered calling down curses instead of blessing them in Christ. So much for praying for your enemies. I'm embarrassed to admit some of my hateful thoughts over the years. Occasionally, when someone hurt me, I wished they would just die. I never did anything to hurt them; I always left that up to God. *Lord, let her get run over by a bus. God, please let aliens abduct him. I don't care how you do it. Just make him disappear from my life.*

Cancer made me angry—barging in on my life, threatening my family and me. Losing control of my life made me angry. The prospect of missing out made me angry. The financial cost of cancer made me angry. Having to go to the appointments, have the scans, take the meds—all of it made me furious. My anger related to cancer dwarfed all the other anger of my life.

Since you can't take out your anger on cancer, I probably took it out on the people around me who loved me the most. I snapped at my family, spoke unkindly at times, and acted impatiently. I withdrew from friends and family. I felt more anger toward those who had hurt me in the past. In some way, everyone made me angry. The guy who pulled out in front of me just as I approached the intersection—*Hey, jerko! Learn how to drive!*

I was on my way out of the post office when my oncologist called. I stopped in the middle of the lobby and listened to some bad news about my recent scans. Unsure what to do next, and lost in my thoughts, I stood there frozen. As people came and went all around me, doors opening and closing, post office boxes being checked, packages and letters being sent and received, I heard God speak to me.

Well, you said you wanted them out of your life. You may just get your wish.

I knew what God meant. The message had been delivered. If cancer killed me, I wouldn't have to see any of the people who had hurt and angered me ever again. Never again would I be frustrated with my wife, my kids, extended family, and friends, coworkers, neighbors, church leaders, or anyone else. Problem solved. I could learn to forgive and get over my anger, or God could take me out of the equation, which would be far easier. The choice was mine.

My hypocrisy could not have been made any clearer if a mailman had plowed his truck through the wall, into the post office lobby, rolled down his window, and handed me the message. God wasn't angry with me. God forgave me. God didn't keep a record of my wrongs, shut me out, wish me harm, or pray I would die. God loved me, no matter what. Jesus had died for me so I could be forgiven and forgiving.

I thought about many of the people I had hurt who somehow forgave me. In every dimension of my life, in every season of my life, I had experienced amazing forgiveness. I thought about the many people I had hurt over the course of my life that I never apologized to, whom I hoped would forgive me.

Thoroughly convicted, I knew I had much repenting and forgiving to do. Clearly, God intended to use my cancer experience as a time to teach me about forgiveness.

The Bible has a lot to say about forgiveness. Over the past twenty years of ministry, I had taught and preached on forgiveness more times than I could count.

Forgiveness begins with God forgiving us. Through faith in Jesus Christ's sacrificial death for us and his resurrection, we are forgiven of our sin and able to have a relationship with God.

It follows naturally, or should we say supernaturally, that we would forgive one another. As we pray in the Lord's prayer, we desire to forgive others as God has forgiven us. Scripture tells us, "We can't love God and hate someone" (1 John 4:20).

"Get rid of all bitterness, rage, and anger, brawling and slander, along with every form of malice. Be kind and compassionate to one another, forgiving each other, just as in Christ God forgave you" (Ephesians 4:31-32).

"Love is patient, love is kind. It does not envy, it does not boast, it is not proud. It does not dishonor others, it is not self-seeking, it is not easily angered, it keeps no record of wrongs. Love does not delight in evil but rejoices with the truth. It always protects, always trusts, always hopes, always perseveres. Love never fails" (1 Corinthians 13:4-8).

I knew all these verses and many others. Still, I struggled to forgive.

I had seen forgiveness at work in the lives of my parishioners. I remember a beloved patriarch of a church I had once served. He was an older man. I will call him Stanley for the sake of confidentiality. He had been diagnosed with an aggressive cancer. Despite a long, intense battle and trying every remedy possible, the end appeared to be imminent. He wanted his family, children, and grandchildren, to come together and pray for healing. He asked me to come to lead them in a healing service at his home.

Stanley confided that lots of conflict existed between his children over disagreements that went years back. They harbored a lot of bitter feelings, anger, and resentment towards each other, and perhaps deep down towards him. Despite living within stone's throw of one another, the siblings hadn't spoken to one another in years. The brokenness grieved him.

Because each one loved their dad, they agreed to come to the healing service the next day. The siblings, their spouses, children, and I crowded into Stanley's living room. Sensing the tension, I quickly started the healing service. I assured them of God's love and promise to heal Stanley. I also explained that God's healing can come in many ways, sometimes not as we most wanted, but the needed healing would come. I read Scripture, said a prayer, and invited them to stand in a circle around their dad and lay their hands on him as we prayed for Stanley. One by one, each sibling prayed aloud for their dad. As they did, I felt their anger subsiding and the walls between them crumbling. Afterward, I anointed Stanley with holy oil, making a cross on his forehead, and praying a final prayer.

As I said goodbye to everyone and took my leave, I watched the siblings embrace one another, Stanley embrace each of them, and then all of them embrace in a big family hug. Smiles, glistening with tears, covered their faces. Although Stanley died a few days later, God had healed his children's relationship that night.

The time had come for me to practice what I preached and stop being angry and start forgiving. Forgiveness was "priority mail" I needed to start delivering immediately. The matter was urgent, "do or die." All the hate mail I had sent God had been rejected and stamped "return to sender." Although removing me from the planet would be easier, God seemed intent to use cancer to cure me of my anger and unforgiveness.

At the time cancer showed up, my marriage stood most in need of forgiveness. Everything Amy did seemed to exasperate me. The way she managed our money, parented our kids, seemingly failed to appreciate anything I did, ignored my needs, and constantly criticized me—it all irked me. And she seemed to be constantly irritated with me, which ironically, made me even more angry. I had become resentful of Amy's attending school to earn her nursing degree instead of earning more income for our family. That lifelong, hard-fought dream of hers was an effort that should have received my full support.

Just a couple of months before my cancer diagnosis, we were preparing to celebrate our twentieth anniversary. I had planned a weekend getaway for us that I now didn't want to go on, but knew we needed. I hoped some time away might relieve some of the pressure and stress. We could both use a fun getaway.

I found a nice gift and a last-minute card. I tried to make it sweeter by including a list of twenty things I loved most about Amy. As we left for the beach, I committed not to talk about things that made me angry so we could have a good time, and we did!

I'll never forget our anniversary dinner, scrounging for loose change in our car so we could have enough money to buy a couple of tacos off the dollar menu at the nearby fast-food restaurant. The next day, we laughed as a gust of wind sent our new multi-colored beach umbrella bouncing down the sandy shore. After Amy's paycheck posted that afternoon, we had a couple of deliciously delightful meals. At one waterfront restaurant, we watched a tugboat pull a massive cargo ship through the harbor while we feasted on seafood and sipped our beach drinks.

On the car ride home, I broke my commitment and said something that conjured up a nor'easter that blew our beach bliss away. We argued all the way home. In the kitchen, as we yelled at each other, Amy threw her gift and card into the trash. I pulled out the card I had given her, with all twenty reasons, ripped it into pieces, and stuffed it back into the trash can. When the kids arrived home, we withdrew in silence to our corners.

The Bible says, "Do not let the sun go down while you are still angry" (Ephesians 4:26). I soon understood why. Having broken that law far too many times, I found myself in a dark place. I felt not only anger but cold-hearted disdain. I started thinking seriously about separation and divorce. My close friends and my counselor tried to pull me back into the light, but I found a way to use their advice to justify my intentions. I told myself I could be a better person, parent, Christian, and even pastor without Amy. I told Amy how I wanted to separate. I felt trapped and angrier than ever.

All that changed when Hurricane Cancer showed up on the horizon, barreling towards us, and then made landfall. We had to be on the same team. Going to medical appointments, processing everything, preparing ourselves for what might lie ahead, calling for help, and comforting our children took all our energy. I had to stop fighting Amy so we could fight together against cancer. Crises have a way of bringing people together.

One night shortly after my diagnosis, I was in bed fast asleep, when out of nowhere, an agonizing pain gripped my side. I tried to lift myself to get out of bed, but the pain in my side drove me back. I tried to roll to my other side, but twisting hurt even more. I laid still, took deep breaths, and worried. *Is this the cancer? What is going on?* Then, by sheer force of will, I swung myself out of bed and onto my feet only to find it hurt just as much to stand. I stood beside the bed, unable to move and on the verge of tears.

Just then, like something out of a superhero movie, Amy jumped up out of bed, threw the blankets off herself, and rushed to my side. Somehow, Super Nurse assessed the problem through my whimpers and moans and comforted me. I probably had bruised a rib or two. She sat me down on the side of the bed and ran downstairs to get me a cup of water and some pain medication. Once back, she arranged my pillows in the perfect way, helped me back into the bed, and tucked the sheets in around me. To top it all off, she gave me a kiss on my forehead. A moment later, she was back in her original spot, fast asleep like nothing happened. Amazing.

As I lay in bed, afraid to move an inch for fear of the pain returning, I thought about Amy. I knew she would be an awesome nurse. I knew something else too—she's a great person, a great mom, a great friend, and a great wife. I thought about how much I loved her and needed her. I wouldn't want to go through this with anyone else. Gratitude for Amy overwhelmed me. I knew I needed to stop being angry and start forgiving. I told her I loved her and that I was sorry. I don't know if she heard me, but I needed to say it. Finally, I fell asleep.

In the morning, during my devotional time, I read the story of God creating Eve. God had already created Adam, but soon realized he needed a partner. "The Lord God said, "It is not good for the man to be alone. I will make a helper suitable for him" (Genesis 2:18). To fix the situation, God created Eve from one of Adam's ribs while he was sleeping. When Adam woke up, he met Eve. The two would be one flesh. Adam would cling to her always.

The story resonated deeply—the long night, the rib connection, and a partner. Once again, I could hear the Lord speaking to me. *David, it's not good for you to be alone. That's why I made Amy for you to be your partner. You are to take care of each other and to work together. You are to cling to her and be one flesh with her. The pain you felt last night is like the pain your anger is causing Amy in her heart. I created you to be forgiving and loving.*

That night saved our marriage. After that, I started letting go of things that made me angry and forgiving her. Letting go is foundational to forgiveness. I let go of my anger about her schooling taking longer than we had expected. I let go of my anger about finances. I let Amy take over them. I let go of the things that so easily offended me—telling me how to drive, not saying thank you, criticizing me. I didn't become a saint, but I was trying, and it felt good.

In my devotional time, I read these words: "You are always and dearly loved by God. So robe yourself with virtues of God....Be merciful as you endeavor to understand others, and be compassionate, showing kindness toward all. Be gentle and humble, unoffendable in your patience with others" (Colossians 3:12 TPT). The call to be unoffendable hit home. I tended to be so easily offended. If I stopped being such a wuss, I wouldn't be angry as much.

Having let go of the anger, I wanted to love her better. I knew acts of service made her feel most loved, so I loaded and unloaded the dishwasher, changed lightbulbs, and helped her with anything she asked—all with renewed vigor and heart. I knew this filled her love tank. As one relationship guru taught, I received these requests as love tags, not nags.

A couple of days later, I did an exercise related to forgiveness that I remembered from a book I had read about marriage. On a piece of paper, I wrote everything about Amy I didn't like, everything that made me angry. When I finished, I ripped the list into shreds as a symbol of my forgiving her once and for all. Next, on a new piece of paper, I wrote everything I loved and appreciated about Amy. That list I would keep with me always and review often.

As I made my list of things I loved, I got an idea too good to be my own. The Holy Spirit must have inspired me. I got a piece of the kids' construction paper the size of a small poster. With a Crayola marker in my hand and tears in my eyes, I wrote on it the twenty things I loved most about Amy. I could remember them just as I had written them on the card I had ripped up and thrown away after our anniversary trip. When I finished, I drew some hearts in the corners and connected them with a squiggly border. At the top, I wrote, "After twenty years of marriage, these are the twenty things I love about you most..." At the bottom, I signed, "Love, David." I had my love poster matted and framed, and gift wrapped and gave it to Amy on her birthday, a few weeks after our anniversary. That remains the best gift I have ever given.

The changes in my relationship with Amy positively impacted my relationships with my family, friends, and life in general. I had grievances I had been holding on to for a long time. I finally let them go. I tried to be forgiving with my kids instead of blowing up whenever they made a wrong move. I tried to be more forgiving daily in everything. Instead of being angry, I wanted to be appreciative of my kids and love them well. When doctors ran behind schedule, which was almost always the case, I tried to be forgiving. Instead of waiting angrily, I tried to wait patiently with an appreciation for my doctors.

The other area in my life most in need of forgiveness was my relationship with the church. Being a pastor had blessed me with some of my life's most wonderful experiences, memories, and friendships. I will forever be grateful. But the church had also been the cause of very painful and disappointing situations.

As God led me to forgive fellow Christians who had hurt me, the story of Joseph (Genesis chapters 37-50) took on special meaning. Joseph's brothers plot to kill him. One of the brothers convinces the others to sell him into slavery instead. They carry out their plan, and soon Joseph is in a dungeon in Egypt, awaiting his fate.

Of course, the story isn't over. God intervenes, and soon Joseph is living and serving in the Pharaoh's house. Impressed by Joseph, the Pharaoh appoints him to be second-in-command over the entire country. When Joseph prophesizes that years of terrible famine are coming, Pharaoh puts him in charge of overseeing the stockpiling of grain for the nation.

Years later, the famine strikes, and Joseph's brothers come to Egypt—the one place known to have grain—desperate for help. In a twist of fate, they stand before Joseph, unaware of his identity, begging for grain. Joseph reveals himself to them. They are overwhelmed with fear and grief. Joseph reassures them of his forgiveness and continued love, and then speaks these famous words: "...God intended it for good to accomplish what is now being done, the saving of many lives" (Genesis 50:20).

I cannot overstate how much those words helped me deal with the pain the church had caused me. It was an epiphany. In each hurtful situation, I could see, whatever had happened and why it happened, that God intended it for good.

God had big plans for my life and would use everything for my good. God was authoring my story, and no one else. The people who hurt me were just minor characters in my story, not authors. God may have led them to do what they did. Or God may have opted to use their error and folly to help fulfill his perfect plans for me. Only God could see the big picture. I could not. All I could do was trust the loving sovereignty of God and his promises. "For I know the plans I have for you," said the LORD, "plans to prosper you and not to harm you, plans to give you hope and a future" (Jeremiah 29:11).

I still felt hurt by the way my last church had let me go, but I knew what I needed to do. Ironically, a few months earlier, I had preached an entire sermon series on conflict. I had devoted one week to the many ways we can respond to being hurt instead of choosing to be angry. I made a point to name several options. Thanks to Jesus, we have the freedom to choose. Instead of being angry, we could let it go, maybe even laugh about it. We could lean in and learn from it. We could leverage the painful experience and let it fuel us to do something good. We could love our enemies as Jesus taught us and pray for them (Matthew 5:44). Of course, we could also choose to forgive.

Joseph's story also helped me reconcile my anger towards God. God allowed cancer to happen to me. God is sovereign. We receive nothing that hasn't passed through God's hands. It's either willed by God or permitted by God. I didn't know why God allowed cancer, but I knew God somehow meant it for good. God isn't filled with contempt towards me. God doesn't hate me. God loves me, is with me, and has good things planned for my life. God uses everything that happens to me for my good.

Having a you-meant-it-for-harm-but-God-meant-it-for-good perspective allowed me to see all my painful experiences in a new light. God had always been in control and always would be. I believed God was using every experience, especially the painful ones, to help me become who he wanted me to be and get me to where he wanted me. I could see God using cancer for my good, using cancer to cure me, to help me become more Christ-like in every dimension of my life. Undoubtedly, that included helping me learn to get over my anger and forgive.

Compassion

The night before my bronchoscopy, Matt, a friend of mine from a few years earlier, messaged me to say he also had stage 4 lung cancer and had been through a similar biopsy. He invited me to call him so he could share his experience with me and encourage me.

Prompted by Matt's message, I remembered hearing a couple of years earlier that he had been diagnosed with lung cancer. Although we had worked together on several projects over a few years and gotten to know each other in the process, I had never reached out to him. I hoped he was doing well, and called, anxious to hear what he had to say.

Matt answered, sounding groggy and disoriented. I felt horrible for possibly waking him up and apologized, but he assured me he was glad I had called and got right to the point.

"David, I had a biopsy early in my cancer journey, too."

I encouraged Matt to tell me all about it, and he continued.

"It was terrible! The doctors stuck long, big needles through my back and side. They had a hard time getting to the tumor, but they kept trying. It hurt like hell. Afterward, I bled out of my mouth, almost uncontrollably. I coughed up blood and had a hard time breathing. The doctors got it under control in a matter of a few minutes. But long story short, my biopsy was a nightmare."

As he spoke, I felt his pain in my side and grimaced. My heart began to race. I thought I might have an anxiety attack and die right then. *Why are you telling me this?*

I expressed my regret that his biopsy had gone so badly, thanked Matt for sharing, and started looking for a way to end the call, but Matt had more to say.

"David, no treatment has been effective for my lung cancer. Now I have a tumor in my brain and another in my leg, and nothing can be done. This past Sunday, I resigned from my job. Now all the doctors can do is try to manage my pain. It's hard to do what I need to do and finish the book I'm writing."

Despite my anxiety being off the charts, I felt overwhelming compassion for Matt. I felt sincere regret for not having reached out to him. As Matt talked, I remembered seeing his many social media posts and hearing from another friend about Matt's cancer. I had known, but I had never acknowledged knowing.

Despite his fatigue, pain, and frustration, he took the time to reach out to me.

"Matt, I'm so sorry you're having such a hard time. How can I help you? What can I do? Please forgive me for not reaching out to you."

With a burst of strength, Matt stopped me. "David, I called to minister to you, not for you to minister to me. I called to encourage you. God's got this. God's got you. God's got your family. God is good. God loves you. God is in control. God is more powerful than cancer. God always makes a way, and God will make a way for you."

To end our call, Matt asked if he could pray for me. Although a little afraid of what he might say, I accepted, and he prayed a beautiful, powerful prayer over my family and me.

Afterward, still feeling Matt's pain in my side, I marveled at his phone call. That he had called, despite his illness and despite never having heard from me, deeply moved me. It also convicted me that I needed to do a much better job of reaching out.

The next morning, as I waited for my bronchoscopy, I sat surrounded by friends and family. Through the crowded room, I saw two women in the hallway headed towards the waiting room. As they came closer, I recognized them as two dear friends, Susan and Ashley. We had become close friends years earlier while I served as their pastor. They and Amy had become like sisters and remained close.

Their visit surprised me and moved me. I felt overcome with emotion upon seeing them. They had driven a long distance to see me. They seemed like angels visiting me. Their love and tenderness touched me deeply. I had to hold back the tears as they embraced Amy and me.

In the days to come, as word of my cancer diagnosis circulated, countless people reached out to me. Cards, messages, prayers, meals, and offers to help came in like a flood. Family, friends, parishioners, colleagues, and strangers reached out. People from every stage of my life from childhood through the present contacted me with concern and good wishes. Many reached out to help me cover medical expenses. Parishioners stopped by my office to offer a word of prayer and encouragement.

Often the acts of kindness and compassion would remind me, like Matt's call had, of times I hadn't reached out.

I vividly remembered driving to work twenty years earlier and passing a car stopped on the side of the road with its hazard lights flashing. The distraught driver stood beside it, waving for someone to help. I drove by without stopping, looking over my shoulder at the poor guy. I can't remember why I didn't stop—if I was running late, or just assumed someone else would stop. Either way, a minute later, I felt painfully convicted, turned the car around, and went back to help. Although only a couple minutes had passed, the vehicle and driver had vanished. God seemed to have put me to the test. I may or may not have failed, but I certainly didn't get an "A."

I thought about my beloved maternal Grandma, who died my second year of undergraduate college. I had been close to her and my grandad. They loved me, and I loved them. I told my mom and dad that I couldn't go to Michigan for the funeral for some reason I've long since forgotten. Instead, I talked to my broken-hearted grandad on the phone for a few minutes. I told him I was sorry. I regret to this day not having gone. Nothing could have been more important.

More than just making me feel guilty and bad about myself, all the acts of compassion I had received since my cancer diagnosis and the memories of the times I had failed to reach out gave me a new appreciation for reaching out and showing compassion. For the first time, I knew how much it meant when someone showed up.

Twenty years of ministry had given me many opportunities to show up for others. While I surely missed some of those as well, I could also recall times when I had been there to offer the compassion of Christ.

I comforted Jessica in the first few hours after learning her husband had been killed in the Iraq war. I ministered to Jude when he was facing imminent death and felt tortured by the guilt of his infidelity decades earlier. I sat in the ER, holding the hand of a teenage boy who had somehow shot himself in the head. I tended to the sick. I prayed with scared and nervous parishioners and their loved ones before and after surgeries. I visited lonely, shut-in seniors. I held the hand of the dying. I ministered to the bereaved and presided over funerals with grace and dignity. I counseled and encouraged couples on the brink of divorce.

As I pondered these and other memories, I had a revelation. Until cancer entered my life, I had not known how much my showing up meant. Once I had been dependent on others showing up for me, I finally got it. After being in need and receiving the compassion of others, I now understood how much my compassion for others meant.

I grieved the pain I had caused Amy, my children, my family and friends, parishioners, and many others I cared about when I hadn't shown up. *I'm sorry, Grandpa. I should have been there for you.*

I grieved the opportunities I had missed, the times I had driven by those in need without stopping. I wondered why I hadn't reached out more. Maybe I had been too busy with work. I hoped I hadn't reached out only when I had to, when my job called for it. I may have been too focused on my world to notice what was happening in anybody else's. Maybe my heart, like the Grinch's, had been "two sizes too small."[4]

A Bible verse I had long known came to mind with new significance. "Praise be to the God and Father of our Lord Jesus Christ, the Father of compassion and the God of all comfort, who comforts us in all our troubles, so that we can comfort those in any trouble with the comfort we ourselves receive from God" (2 Corinthians 1:3-4).

So many had shown me so much compassion that I had been comforted beyond comprehension. Passing on the compassion and comfort I had received would take a lifetime. I felt hopeful that God would use my cancer to make me more compassionate.

I thought of other Bible verses and illustrations about compassion. I had known many of them my whole life. I had preached and taught them. But now, as a cancer patient being cared for, I cared more.

The Bible teaches us that God is compassionate. The Psalmist proclaims, "You Lord, are a compassionate and gracious God, slow to anger, abounding in love and faithfulness" (Psalm 86:15). John assures us that "God is love," and we are loved by God (1 John 4:8).

God's love is shown through compassion. "Because of the Lord's great love, we are not consumed, for his compassions never fail. They are new every morning; great is your faithfulness" (Lamentations 3:22-23).

Jesus Christ is God's incarnate, in-the-flesh, compassion. "For God so loved the world he gave his one and only Son, that whoever believes in him shall not perish but have eternal life" (John 3:16).

With cancer, I needed to be reminded more than ever of God's love for me. I hungered for assurances of God's graciousness and goodness, plans to prosper me, and the promises of daily compassions. These Bible affirmations and promises fed my soul.

Most importantly, the Bible helped me remember Jesus' presence with me through everything. I leaned hard on Jesus. There truly was for me, as the old hymn proclaims, no other way than to trust and obey. When I thought of Jesus, I soon thought of his compassion for me and for all.

"When (Jesus) saw the crowds, he had compassion on them, because they were harassed and helpless, like sheep without a shepherd" (Matthew 9:36).

Jesus reached out to the sick, grieving, the lonely, the marginalized, and all kinds of broken people. Jesus sent his disciples out to do the same. Jesus continues to call Christians to show up and show compassion.

Jesus' sacrificial death for the world is the most potent demonstration of compassion ever and our high calling. "This is how we know what love is: Jesus Christ laid down his life for us. And we ought to lay down our lives for our brothers and sisters" (1 John 3:16).

Since my childhood, I had known the Church's heart of compassion. I had seen the Body of Christ in motion. As a pastor, I had witnessed, time after time, churches being the hands and feet of Christ. Despite each church's flaws, I had witnessed their unmatched commitment to outreach. Within that caring community, I had known many Christians who had devoted themselves to ministries of compassion in ways that continued to inspire me.

I will never forget sitting at a restaurant in Fayetteville, North Carolina, with Dr. Miller and a few other men from our church for a Bible study when news of Hurricane Katrina broke. After seeing the images of the chaos ensuing in New Orleans, he excused himself to make a phone call. When he returned a few minutes later, he announced that he would be leaving that afternoon, flying down to help. In five minutes, he had arranged for a plane, medical supplies, a team to go with him, and a base location in the city. Repeatedly, the good doc dropped everything to answer the cry for help. He was a prominent and successful plastic surgeon by day and a medical missionary by night.

Bryan's passion for prison ministry stood second to none. For years, he had given up every Thursday night to help lead a men's Bible study at the local prison. He knew the inmates' stories, hurts, and hopes. He treated each one with dignity, humility, tenderness, and strength. He invested untold hours into building positive relationships with the warden and other key prison staff. On most Sundays, he signed out a qualifying inmate and brought him to worship with his family and lunch afterward. He spent many weeks each year planning a special annual event that united inmates and their children at our church for a day of faith and family building.

Helen's passion for food ministry captivated me and many others. If an event at our church involved food, she supported it and probably led it. Helen engineered the meal train that fed my family and me for several months. Above all else, Helen's missionary passion was making sure a nearby shelter for battered women had delicious and nutritious food. She cooked for the women like she was cooking for Jesus. She served only the finest meats and freshest vegetables. She worked tirelessly to develop relationships with local food suppliers so the women could eat the best. Often, she joined the women for supper, using the time to get to know them and to tell them how much Jesus loved them.

About six months after my cancer diagnosis, I met Terry, a sixty-two-year-old bachelor diagnosed with pancreatic cancer a few months earlier, at almost the same time as my diagnosis. Terry had the good fortune of having a caring family and a loving sister, Julie, who happened to be a member of my church and one of my favorite people. Since his diagnosis, Julie had kept me updated on his journey, which more recently had included an invasive, complicated surgery that had required a long recovery and left him weakened. Trying to encourage him, Julie told him how well I was doing, shared with him my blog posts about my cancer experience, and tried to use them as an opportunity to talk with her brother about faith in Jesus. She worried about his potential lack of faith and church attendance. She told him about our shared love of guitars and music.

One afternoon, Julie stopped by my office and asked me to go out with her to the parking lot and meet Terry. He was in town to receive his first dose of chemo at the nearby hospital. His care had been transferred there from his home hospital two hours away. We walked out to the SUV, where Terry sat in the front passenger seat, wearing a bright smile and dark sunglasses, which seemed to accentuate his pale white skin and thin face. He reached out through the open window to shake my hand firmly and warmly.

In the few minutes we had together in the church's parking lot, my heart burst for Terry. I encouraged him and committed to helping him in any way possible. I asked if I could pray for him, and he accepted. I took his hand in mine and prayed for him, Julie, and his family. I promised to visit him at the hospital.

After Terry's first chemotherapy treatment, his health went from bad to worse, and after a couple of days at home, he was back in town and in the hospital with a bleak prognosis. In the days to follow, he developed a severe infection that damaged his kidneys, created other complications, and prevented any more treatments. Meanwhile, the cancer continued to spread like wildfire.

I continued to visit Terry often, motivated by my love for Julie and my deepening connection with Terry. I felt a great sense of unfairness as everything seemed to go so well for me while Terry couldn't get a break.

In our visits, we talked about guitars, music, work, family, and hobbies. I also looked for an opportunity to talk about his relationship with Jesus Christ, longing to make sure he had one.

One day, as I visited, Terry confessed the intense difficulty of needing so much help from Julie and his mom. He had always been responsible for helping others. I assured him it was okay to need help. I tried to explain to Terry that letting his family help him was a great gift to them. They wanted to and needed to help. They all nodded as they wiped the tears from their eyes and thanked him for letting them love him and be there for him.

I recognized my opening to talk about faith in Jesus, the urgency of time, and gave it my best.

"Terry, the truth is that we all need help, just like we need God's help. So many things are beyond our power. We need God to be forgiven, to have a good relationship with him and our loved ones. We need God to become more like Jesus, to be healed, to have strength, hope, and eternal life. We can't do anything on our own. God helps us through his Son, Jesus Christ, when we put our faith in him. The Bible says that we are saved by grace through faith in Jesus, not by works."

Terry nodded, clearly moved by the conversation. With that, I took Terry's hand in my own and prayed for him, his faith in Jesus, and his eternal salvation. I praised God for him and his faith in Jesus.

The next day, my phone rang while Amy and I were having dinner at a nearby restaurant. I recognized Julie's number and answered. I heard her try to speak, and then the phone went silent, and the call ended. She texted me a minute later to confirm my fears. "He's leaving us tonight." Another text followed. "Please come ASAP and bring your guitar if possible. Terry would like you to play and sing some songs."

Because the cold I had been fighting for the last few days had gotten much worse first since my previous visit with Terry, I questioned if my going was a good idea. Amy pointed out my flawed thinking; germs didn't matter at this point. She insisted I go immediately. I texted back that I was on my way, raced to my house, picked up my guitar, took a double dose of cold medicine, and sped to the hospital.

As I entered the room, Terry's gaze fixed on the guitar case. As I unpacked the guitar and music, Julie introduced me again to her mom, sister, and one of her brothers. I told Terry how sorry I was to hear the doctor's bleak report, and asked if he would like to listen to some songs. He thanked me and nodded.

I sang "Amazing Grace," and the family joined joined their voices with mine. I reminded Terry of how we are all saved by grace, in need of God's help, and he smiled. I sang a song about God's unconditional love. Halfway through, my nose started to run, my eyes began to water, and my throat became scratchy. I felt hot and cold and started sweating profusely. I wiped the sweat off my head with my sleeve and pressed on with one last song about God razing Lazarus from the dead. I assured Terry that Jesus had a special place for him in heaven.

I sensed the time had come for me to leave. Terry looked tired. I wanted to give the family time alone with him. After I packed up my guitar and music, I took Terry's hand in mine and leaned towards him. I looked into his eyes and said, "Terry, I believe you are trusting in Jesus. If you are, you know that everything is going to be okay. You don't need to be afraid. Jesus has a place in heaven for you. Great things are in store for you. Terry, do you believe in Jesus?"

With no hesitation, Terry looked me in the eyes and replied, "Yes, I do."

Inviting everyone to clasp hands and circle around Terry's hospital bed, I prayed one last time with Terry.

Terry died peacefully the next day, in hospice, in Julie's arms, surrounded by his family.

I presided over Terry's funeral in his hometown. I played Terry's favorite guitar and sang "Amazing Grace" for his grieving family and friends. In my message, I shared some of his story and his faith in Jesus Christ. After the service, a man approached me with tears in his eyes and a smile on his face and hugged me. He and Terry had been best friends since childhood. While Terry's friend had decided to become a Christian and put his faith in Jesus many years ago, as far as he knew, Terry never had. Terry's suspected lack of faith grieved his friend terribly, especially when he heard Terry had died. To know that Terry believed in Jesus Christ gave him overwhelming joy. He thanked me and embraced me again.

I knew my ministry to Terry was important to him and his family. I knew it was also important to me, but I had no idea how much it would change my life. When I stepped into Terry's life, I took my first steps toward a new calling from God to minister to those suffering from cancer. I had never had an outreach passion like Matt, Mark, Bryan, Helen, until I met Terry. For nearly twenty years, my mission had been the church in general. That all changed when I met Terry.

Now I felt a desire to reach out to cancer patients and their families. As I came in and out of the hospital and clinics, I saw them with their ports, IVs, bandages, hats, and scarves to cover their baldness. I saw them, my fellow cancered ones. I saw their fatigue, worry, and fear. I saw their wheelchairs and walkers. I saw them searching for a parking place and trying to be on time. I watched as they waited too long for the doctors to see them. I overheard the hospital representatives going over insurance and finance matters with them. I could feel my heart breaking for all the cancer patients and their loved ones.

My continued good reports and progress reminded me of those not getting similar reports and struggling. I thought of those I had known and loved who also had cancer. I remembered my mother-in-law, the surgeries she'd endured, the little "barf bucket" that always accompanied her. I knew what they were going through. I wanted to help, advocate, and make a difference.

I didn't know what my outreach to the cancered ones would look like exactly, but I did know that like God called Paul to the gentiles, God had called me to reach out with compassion to those facing cancer. I started writing this book in the hope that it would one day provide insight, guidance, and inspiration to those enduring cancer.

How amazing! God had been using my cancer all along to help me become more compassionate. I had come to expect that God would continue that work in me, but I was surprised when he called me into a ministry to cancer patients, survivors, and their families. What better way for me to continue growing to become a more compassionate human being.

As I finished this chapter, I could hear some of the songs I had sung at the conclusion of countless worship services as the congregation and I were sent out into the world, songs about hearing God calling us to serve those in need, and hymns about our hearts overflowing with compassion. I could still feel God tugging on my heart.

Get-Up-And-Go

The day came for us to move our oldest daughter, Marcie, into college for the first semester of her freshman year. We all had been looking forward to it. I felt proud that she had chosen my alma mater, Appalachian State University, in beautiful Boone, North Carolina. I had been praising God for enabling us to find the money for her to go. I always enjoyed going up to the mountains. This would be an extra special trip, and the weather forecast looked great.

But now I didn't want to go. With the doctor's pronouncement of doom ringing in my ears—"It's cancer"—I couldn't imagine being able to enjoy this trip, or even pretending to enjoy it. I felt depressed, sorry for myself, and angry at the world. I couldn't bear the thought of a three-hour drive with all these morbid thoughts rolling through my mind.

I thought about pretending to be sick. I could fake an emergency at work. Amy and the kids could handle this without me. Amy could drive her. We couldn't fit all of Marcie's stuff in the SUV, plus the five of us, anyway. My staying home would give them more precious room.

Our struggle to pack the SUV blew up into a full-blown conflict with yelling, screaming, tears, and with mother and daughter arguing. *I need that. No, you don't. We will bring it to you. I need it now. This won't fit. Yes, it will...if you pack it like this.*

You can't pack it that way. My attempt to intervene only added gasoline to the fire.

The escalating drama confirmed my desire to stay home. Just as the words were about to come out of my mouth, Amy said she would *not* be going. "Your dad can take you!" she yelled as she stormed into the house and slammed the door behind her. Now, not only would I have to go, I would somehow have to convince Amy to go, too!

On the three-hour drive, Amy slept, and the kids listened to music with the earphones. I had plenty of time to think. *Will I be alive to move her out in the summer? Will I get sick during the semester? How aggressive is this cancer? Will I distract her and cause her to not do well? Will I see her graduate? Will I see her get married?* The thoughts kept coming.

We arrived at the dormitory and pulled into the chaotic sea of vehicles, patrolled by orange-vested traffic guides efficiently directing students and parents. Miraculously, within a matter of minutes, we had transported all of Marcie's belongings to the sixth floor of the dorm and into the tiny shoebox room with two of everything and zero air conditioning.

The carpet the roommates had chosen for their room was too big and wouldn't work. Marcie's roommate, distressed over the matter, was letting her dad have it.

I backed out of the overcrowded, hot-as-Hades room and into the hall, stood by the doorway, and watched the two girls, their moms, their siblings, and the roommate's dad set up the room. I felt sad and out of place. I wanted to crawl into one of the unpacked boxes and hide. Or better yet, be rolled up in the carpet that didn't fit and go wherever it was bound.

Amy and the other mom feverishly wiped everything down with sanitizer. They gave instructions and unpacked boxes. The siblings tried to make the beds while being on top of them. The other dad determinedly hung pictures and lights on the wall, trying to make up for the carpet burn.

As I stood watching, the realization of how quickly the past eighteen years had gone by hit me like a kick in the gut. I couldn't breathe. Life really had gone fast. I hadn't done enough. I should have spent more time with her. There were conversations we should have had. Now my chance had passed.

As my thoughts spun out of control, I felt the presence of Jesus. It was as if he had walked up the hallway, stopped, and put his arm around me, and we watched Marcie together. I could sense Jesus speaking to me.

David, let me tell you what I see. Marcie is an amazing young woman. She's going to be just fine. You're a great dad. You have done a good job. And you still have time to do more. Enjoy today. Keep going.

Just like that, everything started coming into focus. As I watched Marcie trying to stick her string of lights to the wall perfectly, I felt overwhelmed with pride and gratitude. She had grown into an amazing young woman—smart, friendly, faithful, gifted, talented, and beautiful—despite my many shortcomings. She would be successful in school and in life. Ms. Marcie would be a great elementary school teacher.

On our drive home, I felt glad that I had come instead of staying home for my pity party. As I reflected, I had an epiphany. Because of my looming cancer diagnosis, I had enjoyed the day more than I would have otherwise. Cancer wanted me to stop, but God wanted me to keep going. Because of the uncertainty cancer had brought into my life, including the real threat of dying much sooner than I had ever considered, I had treasured the day and my daughter in a way I know I would not have otherwise. Once I got out of my pit of despair, I had thrown myself into the day like never before—fully present, fully engaged, and fully joyful.

I needed to keep going for Marcie, Hannah, Caleb, Amy, and me. After that weekend, I tried hard to cherish each day I had with all three of my children. I hadn't always lived that way. I had taken many things for granted. At times, I had acted like my kids weren't important. On other occasions, I had treated their activities as just one more thing tacked on to an already long workday. Now I didn't want to miss any concert, play, event, or a single moment. I excused myself from work so I could arrive early. I took pictures and made videos of everything, breaking copyright laws left and right, and embarrassing my kids.

I'm sure each person who receives a cancer diagnosis responds differently. I imagine there are some who make a bucket list and get going on it right away. The next week, they're sky diving or skiing in the Alps. The week after that, they're climbing Mount Kilimanjaro. They hop in the car and go reconcile with siblings and friends, burying the hatchet once and for all. For them, cancer is a call to action. It's now or never.

That was not my case. Initially, I didn't want to do anything or go anywhere. Sitting and sulking sounded good to me. Despite my desire to keep going, and how much Marcie's move-in weekend had meant to me, my newfound appreciation for all my kids' activities, and my desire not to miss anything, cancer had taken the wind out of my sails. I felt like my get-up-and-go had got up and left.

As I lamented my sudden lack of vigor and zest for life, it occurred to me that perhaps my get-up-and-go had long been gone. Had I been truly living? Had I appreciated and grabbed hold of the promise of each day? Had I made the most of every moment? When did I last seize the day? Cancer might be more of a call to live than I had first thought.

Over the course of our marriage, Amy had often accused me of never wanting to go anywhere or do anything. I hated hearing that and objected to her exaggeration. But now that cancer had stopped me, I could see and hear myself.

Do you want to go out to dinner? No. Do you want to run some errands and go shopping with me? No. Do you want to visit your parents? No. Do you want to go on a walk with me? No. Do you want to go get your car fixed? No. Do you want to come with me to my friend's wedding? No. Do you want to go on a cruise? I found a killer deal. No. Do you want to go and have that life-threatening cough checked out? No!

It wasn't just with Amy. As I reflected, I could see many times in recent years when I had not wanted to go. I'm sorry to admit that I hadn't always wanted to go to my kid's school performances and conferences. When it came to work, as much I loved being a pastor, there had been times when I loathed going to an important meeting. I didn't want to go to the gym and exercise as much as I needed. I hadn't wanted to go for a run even when the weather was perfect. I had not wanted to go visit my family in Michigan, blaming the cost of airfare or the long drive.

I don't know what had held me back. Maybe I hadn't valued the people in my life enough. Maybe I had taken life for granted. Maybe I assumed there would always be tomorrow. Maybe I had not appreciated my life and my family enough? Maybe I focused too much on myself. Maybe I gave too much of myself to work.

All of these were possibilities. One thing was for sure—I had disappointed a lot of people and missed out on what would have been special times for them and for me. I felt deep regret over what could have been.

I knew that Jesus wanted me to get up and go. My internet search showed Jesus having said the word *go* about a hundred and fifty times. Go and sin no more. Go tell others. Go show yourself. Go, and your son will live. Go make disciples. Go. Go. Go.

Jesus said, "I have come that they may have life, and have it to the full" (John 10:10). I think he meant more than a life full of peace, hope, and love. Jesus came so our lives also could be full of adventure, experiences, surprises, and amazing memories. Jesus came so we might live a full-throttled life. Because of him, we are forgiven and free to push down on the gas, to rev our engine, listen to it roar, put this baby in gear, and go!

I felt confident that God had already started to use cancer to heal me of my lethargy, my inertia, my lack of zest for living, my failure to carpe diem, or whatever you want to call it and give me some get-up-and-go. My cancer diagnosis had provided a much-needed kick in the rear. God used it to spur me back into action and restore my drive.

A few days after the weekend trip with Marcie, I went in for a scan of my chest. My oncologist wanted more images of my lungs and to make sure cancer hadn't spread to my brain. I made jokes with the nurses to calm my nerves. It was my first MRI.

I looked at the poster on the wall across from me as the nurse slid the needle into my arm and started the IV. The poster proclaimed, "Life is full of little pricks," and pictured an actress, famed for her mean character on a popular tv show, dressed as a nurse, smiling slyly and holding a disturbingly large needle in her hand.

A few minutes later, I laid back on the narrow exam table protruding from what looked like a ten-foot-wide silver donut standing vertically. The technicians explained that the procedure would involve a series of scans of varying lengths, from my waste to the top of my head, loud knocking sounds and buzzing, and the injection of the magnetic dye into my arm at the halfway point. The technician put a pair of headphones on me to help lessen the noise and to allow them to speak to me, gave a thumbs-up, and returned to the control room ten feet away.

Through my headphones, she said, "This first scan will take three minutes," and the table began sliding into the doughnut hole.

I gave her the thumbs-up and watched her in the control room, push a series of buttons. "Let's go!" I heard her say, and the knocking and buzzing began.

Her "Let's go!" surprised me, and I thought about it as I laid there. *Let's go. Where am I going? I'm flat on my back, strapped to this table, having an MRI. I've been diagnosed with stage four lung cancer. Hopefully, it's not spread to my brain. This is my fourth scan in three weeks. With each report, the diagnosis worsens. Let's go?*

The first scan ended, and the tech said, "Are you okay?" I gave the thumbs up and smiled. She introduced the next scan. "Okay, this scan will take five minutes. Let's go!"

For the next three minutes, as I felt the vibrations and listened to the knocking, humming, and clanking, "Let's go!" echoed in my mind. The words began to sound like God calling me to move forward into a promising future. *Let's go, David. I have plans for you. This cancer isn't the end for you. It's the beginning. It's not a death sentence. It's a call to live.*

I thought of one of my favorite Bible verses, "I know the plans I have for you," says the Lord, "plans to prosper you and not to harm you, plans to give you hope and a future" (Jeremiah 29:11).

Several more scans ensued, each one launched with the same words, *Let's go...Let's go...Let's go.* It was like a liturgical response in worship. Lord, in your mercy, *hear our prayer.*

During the remaining scans, I thought of things I needed to do, wanted to do, but had not done. Write a book, speak out for justice, be a better husband and father, spend more time with family and friends, and be a more faithful Christian. I thought of changes I needed to make and people I needed to forgive. After each scan, the tech's next "Let's go" seemed to affirm my plans.

The technician told me the final remaining scans would be of my brain. "Are you okay?" she said. "Any questions?"

I gave her the thumbs up and replied, "Let's go!"

Over the course of my lifetime, God had put many people with terrific get-up-and-go in my life to inspire me. A few came to mind.

My dad's get-up-and-go is off the charts. The man never stops. When he worked at Ford Motor Company's factory as a teenager to earn money for college, his fellow linesmen tried to sabotage his assembly line because he was going too fast and making them all look bad. When I was a kid, he worked his way up to the top of the corporate world and then came home and worked non-stop on our house and a fourteen-acre property. He finished a bedroom addition one day and started on a full-size barn the next.

I could see him now, speed-walking through his 54,000-square-foot manufacturing plant, keeping tabs on all the work.

I thought of Matt, a friend and ministry colleague. He started a church with just himself, his wife, and two kids. He then grew it to be a multi-site church worshipping several hundred people every Sunday. I would see pictures on social media of his church in action one day, and then pictures of him on an African safari the next day.

Many parishioners came to mind, too, from hardworking farmers to successful professionals like Dr. Miller. In addition to being a successful plastic surgeon, he made missionary trips multiple times each year, traveled the world, had a great family life, served as a leader in the community and the church, and still found the time and energy to try out to be a contestant on the hit TV show *Survivor*. Each Sunday, I had the opportunity to preach, Dr. Miller left, on the pulpit, an index card for me upon which he had written "Carpe Diem!"

A day after the MRI, my dad invited me to fly with him, my brothers, and my mom to Michigan for my uncle Richard's funeral. My dad would buy the tickets and cover all the expenses. We'd fly up early and come back late the same day. Despite the short notice, nothing stood in my way. All I had to do was go.

I thought I'd like to go despite not having been close to my uncle. My family moved from Michigan to North Carolina when I was ten. I would enjoy seeing my cousins and other extended family. I hadn't been up there in years, and I didn't know when or if I would have another chance. I was touched by my dad's offer. I liked the idea of spending time with him and my family.

Despite these and other reasons to go, I told my dad I didn't think I should. So much for *Let's go!* I was expecting a call from my oncologist to tell me about the treatment options. Although my oncologist encouraged me to go and promised he would call me ASAP with the information, I still wanted to be at home, feet on the ground, ready to go when he called. I didn't want to risk catching a cold or something worse on the airplane. I also worried that between my uncle's death and my disease, the trip could become sad and morbid.

On my way to an appointment later that day, a sports car passed me and cut in front of me just as the light turned red. Inching up, I admired the car's curves, color, the sound of the engine, the twin mufflers, and everything about it. As I oohed and aahed, I noticed the custom license plate: DIELIVING. As I sat idling, staring at the words, which seemed to be getting bigger and bigger, scenes replayed in my mind like a movie montage. I could see and hear them vividly.

The MRI technician announcing, "Let's go. Let's go."

Amy decrying, "You never want to go anywhere or do anything. Just go!"

My dad inviting me. "All you have to do is go."

My oncologist assuring me it was fine for me to travel. "Go. I'll call you ASAP."

Along with the voice of God, they all declared, in unity, "Gooooo!"

A couple of days later, my mom, dad, brothers, and I rendezvoused at 4:00 a.m. for our five o'clock flight. After checking in, we headed down the long concourse to the American Airlines hub, our rolling carry-on bags in tow. Armed with coffee and our cell phones, watches synchronized, we were ready for our mission, which I had chosen to accept. Minutes later, we were taxing into position and then barreling down the runway. Take off!

A few hours later, we pulled out of the rental lot in a minivan. It felt like the old days. My two brothers and I couldn't resist.

"How much longer, Mom? "

"Are we there yet?"

"I've got to pee, Dad."

Off we went to the "cute bungalow" my mom had booked online. We planned to check in and drop off our luggage before heading to lunch. The price was great, a "real steal," which helped since the airplane tickets had cost "an arm and a leg."

The van got quiet as the scenery and streetscape began to look more and more rundown and ghettoish. Every block or two, a neon flashing sign advertising cash advances, liquor, and cigarettes topped another convenience store. Boarded-up houses filled in the rest. We arrived at our street and slowly turned the corner.

"Mom? What did you do?" my younger brother said, with concern in his voice.

From inside the van, we watched my mom and dad check us into the "cute bungalow." They stood on the small front porch with the landlord, who looked nice and harmless. I wondered if "real steal" may have referred to the bars over the windows. A pit bull strolled out from behind the house, dragging his chain behind him. He stopped, turned his head, and looked at us, and then trotted across the yard and took off down the street.

I decided to go in and have a quick tour with my parents. It was clean and furnished comfortably. It would be okay, even with the creepy basement, but we would keep our luggage with us. Although we planned to come back after dark and spend the night, we hurried out of the driveway as fast as we could.

Despite the laughter and jokes, I had never in my life felt more appreciative of my family experience. We had always lived in nice homes and nice neighborhoods. We had two loving parents who had provided us with everything we needed. Going back and spending the night in the cute bungalow would be good for us all.

We headed to my Uncle George and Aunt Sharon's (my dad's sister) high-rise condo in uptown, Detroit. Talk about a tale of two cities. George's bear hug alone made the trip. As a kid, I had looked forward to his hug every summer at the end of our long drive from North Carolina to visit. My aunt gave me a quick peck on the lips. They boarded the minivan, and we were off again to lunch. And afterward, a tour of the city.

My uncle, a lifelong champion of the City of Detroit, worked as a professional tour guide. Unfortunately, his tour was no match for the deep-dish pizza and Canadian beer. I could not keep my eyes open. After fifteen minutes, they mercifully took me back to the condo so I could nap while my aunt prepared dinner. "You need to take care of yourself," she said, as she showed me to the guest room.

After everyone had enjoyed a few hours in the city while I napped, we all reunited at my aunt and uncle's place for more catching up and a wonderful dinner and dessert. Afterward, my family and I headed back to our little bungalow.

We survived the night, and in the morning headed to the funeral. Entering the sanctuary reminded me that Richard had two families—the one from his first marriage, and another from his second. The children from his first marriage and their families with a few friends sat on the right, alone or in little groups, spread out with plenty of space between them. The children of his second marriage and their extended family and friends had to squeeze together into the pews on the other side.

Richard's first marriage had reportedly been a painful and rocky one. Somehow the two managed to raise four great kids, who were young adults by the time their mom and dad split. They all went on to do well and have their own families.

Richard remarried years later, adopted his new wife's two young kids, and became a beloved member of a big extended family. Over the years, his second family saw the addition of grandchildren. It seemed to be a happy, loving marriage. But as often happens, the second marriage commanded most of his time and attention, a reality that I suspected made the funeral more painful for my cousins and their families.

During the funeral, the pastor highlighted the disparity by standing in front of the side of the sanctuary belonging to Richard's second marriage for the entirety of the service. Almost all of the pastor's remarks, stories, and memories shared, even his eye contact, were directed at that side.

After he had finished, the pastor invited members of the congregation to stand and share a memory about Richard. Being a pastor, I had seen this coming and had scribbled a few notes onto the program. I introduced myself as his *first* nephew from his *first* marriage and acknowledged his *first* family. Directing my remarks to my cousins, I expressed gratitude for Richard, my cousins, and their families. I read a passage of Scripture reminiscent of my uncle's love for boating: Jesus calming the storm. I acknowledged their loss, pain, and grief, and assured them of Jesus' presence and love. Jesus had calmed the storm for their dad and welcomed him into the safe harbor of heaven. He would calm their storms, too. I sat down, feeling grateful for the chance to have given the original family a moment of their own pastoral care.

After the funeral and the reception that followed, we loaded back into the minivan and headed to my cousin Mark's house for a wake for Richard's first family and friends. An hour later, we were off again and headed back to the airport.

On our flight home a couple of hours later, I thought about how, at first, I hadn't wanted to go. I was glad I hadn't given in to that temptation. I wouldn't have wanted to miss one second. I loved it all. I marveled at yet another way God was using lung cancer to change me—curing me of my tendency to give up and giving me more get-up-and-go. As we jetted home, I recalled a familiar Bible verse that now meant more than ever. "I press on toward the goal to win the prize for which God has called me heavenward in Christ Jesus" (Philippians 3:14).

In the weeks and months to follow, I lived life with renewed get-up-and-go, determined to seize the day. If I was invited, I generally wanted to go. From the depths of my being, rose a resounding, "Let's go!"

Strength

"You have very thick skin," the doctor said as she made a tiny incision in my neck for the biopsy. "You can't feel me cutting you, can you?" If I had, I would have been running away from the hospital by now, but I appreciated her asking.

As I held my breath and waited, she said again, "Wow! Your skin is very thick, very tough." I could feel her pushing on me. "I'm not sure I've ever seen skin this thick." I could see the determined focus in her eyes.

Starting to feel a little guilty, I responded facetiously, "I'm sorry. As a pastor, I've been criticized a lot. I guess it's given me a thick skin."

"Well, it must be working. Your skin is *very* thick."

I felt the doctor push the guide needle through the incision in my "thick neck." Using ultrasound imaging, she positioned the needle over my super clavicular lymph node. A minute later, out of the corner of my eye, I saw a second needle at least sixteen inches long slide into the end of the first needle, the end of which now rested only millimeters from my trachea.

I looked away. The doctor counted down from three, and I heard the popping sound as she cut the biopsy sample, and then a quick suction sound as she drew the tissue out. She repeated the process several times. One by one, the assistant at her side took the extracted tissue samples down the hall to the pathology lab for testing. They planned to keep me on the table and continue taking and sampling biopsies until pathology confirmed they had what they needed.

As I laid there waiting, I still couldn't believe that the first biopsy, the bronchoscopy, had not been successful. After all the effort and expense, the pulmonologist had failed to retrieve the tissue samples from the tumor required for the pathology studies. In short, the procedure had been a bust.

Fortunately for me, the cancer had spread to a few other locations in my body, one of those being my super clavicular lymph node. Super, indeed. My oncologist, certain it was the same cancer as that in my lung, had ordered a biopsy of the node. It was an easier procedure, a short in-and-out procedure that would only take one or two hours, but still a pain in the neck.

"You have thick skin," the doctor said again. This time I thought of the irony of her words. Generally, I considered myself more thin-skinned than thick-skinned. I tended to worry too much about what others think. I wanted to please others. Criticism hurt. My insecurity had kept me from doing many things I should have. I would have considered my lack of thick skin, one of my most significant weaknesses.

As I laid there looking like Frankenstein with metal tubes jammed in my neck, listening to the popping and sucking sounds of the biopsy, I closed my eyes. I imagined all the ways God could use my cancer to thicken my skin and make me stronger when it came to receiving criticism. That might be another way God used cancer to cure me. God could use cancer to toughen me up as a person and make me stronger. Facing cancer, I needed all the strength I could get.

Just when I thought we were finished, the pathologist returned. She needed more tissue. The doctor reassured me that the anesthesia would last. The popping and sucking sounds continued, along with the pushing and pulling. In all, the doctor made twelve passes and took twelve samples.

I left the hospital feeling relieved and grateful that the procedure had been a success. I felt proud of myself for getting through it, and, if I dare say so, a little bit stronger.

For most of my life, I had considered myself a strong person. I was never Arnold Schwarzenegger strong, but physically I had always been strong and healthy. I could see the workout bench and free weights in the basement of my childhood home, where I worked out as a high schooler. As an adult, I had been active, belonging to several gyms and running often.

I had been strong in other ways, too. I grew up with a dedicated work ethic. I had a persistent resolve, effective communication, well-respected leadership and people skills, and a committed faith. Life had knocked me down a time or two, but I had always gotten back up. For the most part, I had accomplished the things I had set out to do.

Despite all of that, when I was diagnosed with cancer, I didn't feel strong at all. I felt weak. I felt like I had been sacked by a six-hundred-pound linebacker. Lying on my back, with the wind knocked out of me, I wasn't sure I had the strength to get up. To fight cancer, to undergo chemotherapy, surgical biopsies, repeated scans and results, and getting sick—it all felt way too hard. Even with my faith, I felt weak and powerless.

Cancer proved to be a difficult and draining struggle— driving to the hospital, walking from the parking deck to the clinic, waiting for appointments and for my doctor to see me, lying still for the CT scan, having my blood drawn for the umpteenth time, and checking out and getting out of the parking deck. The entire cancer regimen exhausted my strength.

The first few weeks with cancer had been the most difficult of my life. I believed Jesus would heal me, but it was still incredibly hard. It took immense energy and determination every day to not fall into the pit of despair. Waiting for results from scans was awful. I knew the scans could just as easily show that the cancer had grown. Recently, a young man who belonged to our church family had died only a few weeks after being diagnosed with cancer. Putting on a brave face for my family and my church exhausted all my strength.

The diagnosis of cancer reaffirmed and revealed my innate weakness. My strength and power were not enough. Cancer is not a pull-yourself-up-by-your-bootstraps thing. I needed God's strength at work in me to an extent I had never experienced before, only read about. I needed God's cancer-crushing, disease-destroying, life-giving strength.

God faithfully ministers to us wherever we are, and knows what we need. In the first few days and weeks of having cancer, many of the Scripture verses I read were about strength.

"God is our refuge and strength, an ever-present help in trouble" (Psalm 46:1-3).

"Those who hope in the Lord will renew their strength. They will soar on wings like eagles" (Isaiah 40:31).

I knew that God wanted me to be strong. I heard the Lord's command to Joshua and the Israelites echoing in my ears. "Have I not commanded you? Be strong and courageous" (Joshua 1:9).

The Bible reminded me often that God is strong. Our God is a mighty God who strengthens his children.

I heard God's promise that his strength would be more than enough, even for cancer. The same assurance Jesus had given Paul in his difficulties, he now gave me: "My grace is sufficient for you, for my power is made perfect in weakness" (2 Corinthians 12:9).

I knew, with faith in Jesus, I had the strength to face any foe. The Bible proclaims, "I can do all this through him who gives me strength" (Philippians 4:13). Over the years, I had often rhetorically asked my congregation as I preached on this verse, "Does the verse say, 'some things or certain things or the easy things…?' No, the Bible says all things!"

I knew all of this. I had taught and preached it for twenty years. I had experienced God's strength working within me too many times, even to count. God's power alone made it possible for me to preach at my mother-in-law's funeral, to be with parents as their infant child prepared to die, to continue in ministry after failing my first attempt at ordination, to sit with a couple in their fractured marriage, to move on to a new church and lead with excitement after having been painfully let go from the previous church. I knew firsthand the empowering reality of God. I could have done none of this without God.

Despite all that, I still felt overwhelmed and outmatched. I needed God to give me the strength I needed to get up and battle cancer. I needed a strength far greater than my own. I needed to give up on any notion of doing this without God's supernatural empowerment.

One morning, I sat down on the sofa with a cup of coffee in my hand and began my morning meditation.

After some time, the word *strength* settled in my mind and pushed out the rest. I said it several times, breathing in the word *strength*, and then breathing it out.

As I meditated, I thought of Peter and John's encounter with a man with crippled feet. He was begging for money and had given up on ever being physically healed. The disciples didn't have money to give, but they offered to provide him with something even better.

"Peter said, 'I don't have money, but I'll give you this— by the power of the name of Jesus Christ of Nazareth, stand up and walk!' Peter held out his right hand to the crippled man. As he pulled the man to his feet, suddenly, power surged into his crippled feet and ankles. The man jumped up, stood there for a moment, stunned, and then started walking. As he went into the temple courts with Peter and John, he leapt for joy and shouted praises to God" (Acts 3:6-9, TPT).

The whole incident captivated me—the disciples' authority to heal in the name of Jesus, the crippled man now stunned and standing on his feet, then jumping and dancing around town. What intrigued me most was how "power surged" through his body.

I felt immense hope and excitement that Christ's power would surge through me, blasting the cancer out of my body, and energizing my whole being.

I had faith that God would give me the strength needed for the cancer battle. I also believed that God would dramatically increase my understanding of his power. I could experience a force beyond my imagination. I felt certain God would use cancer to make me stronger for cancer and for life.

As I continued to search the Scripture for strength, God put on my heart the Bible's story about Jacob wrestling with God in Genesis 32. The night before Jacob plans to meet with his bitterly estranged brother and hopefully make peace, "a man" attacks him in the dark. During the struggle, the man asks Jacob to let him go. Jacob responds, "I won't let go until you bless me" (verse 26).

The man finally gives up on overpowering Jacob and blesses him. Also, he gives him a new name. "Your name will no longer be Jacob, but Israel, because you have struggled with God and with humans and have overcome" (Genesis 32:28). As a final parting gift, the man gives Jacob an injured hip and a permanent limp.

"The man" is considered by most Bible interpreters to represent God. The struggle may have been literal hand-to-hand combat, or it may have been a spiritual battle. Either way, it can represent our struggles with life and with God. To be "blessed" is to receive God's favor, along with his special gifts, benefits, and opportunities. In my wrestling with cancer, this story connected with me.

I wanted complete physical healing. But more than that, I wanted to be like Jacob, wrestling with God through this ordeal and refusing to let go of God and the cancer until God blessed me. I demanded that God bless me, my wife, our marriage, our children, our family and friends, my church, and every facet of my life. Every day, I wanted to declare to God, "I won't let go until you bless me." I wanted Jacob-like determination and strength.

Jacob gave me an excellent way to approach the cancer battle, a boost of strength, and a little moxie. I refused to let cancer bully me. I wanted to grab hold of it and demand that it bless me and everyone around me. I wanted to make cancer work for me. I claimed that I would emerge from this struggle better and blessed.

That weekend, two of our best friends, Chris and Lynn, drove in from out of town to visit Amy and me. We had been friends for more than ten years, and our families had spent lots of time together. Over the years, Chris and I had become like brothers as we journeyed together through challenging times, confided in one another, and supported each other. Seeing them gladdened my heart.

Saturday, God blessed us with perfect weather, and we decided to go out for a run together. We all liked to run. Chris and Lynn were athletic and always in great shape. I looked forward to introducing them to the network of beautiful trails through the woods that surrounded our neighborhood. We suited up, stretched out, and hit the trail.

Wanting the run to be good for them, I started at a pace significantly faster than I usually would run and chose the most challenging trail, one with many hills and long, steep inclines. About halfway up the second incline, an ascent that seemed to go on forever, I started to regret my hurried pace.

As we finally approached the crest of the hill, I heard Chris tell Lynn, "his breathing sounds good." Not winded at all, Lynn responded, "Yeh, his lungs sound great."

Truthfully, I was hurting. I'm sure they *could* hear my breathing. But their words gave me a boost. From someplace deep inside me, I shouted, "Cancer, you can kiss my...!" I accelerated, left them in the dust, and crested the hill at breakneck speed. Once over the top, I eased off the accelerator so my friends could catch up.

I felt stronger than ever. I ran like I had something to prove. *I can do this. Cancer won't stop me.* I ran for God. *I will "Run in such a way as to get the prize"* (1 Corinthians 9:24).

I had been a runner, although never consistent, for nearly twenty years. With the advent of cancer, I found a new appreciation for running. Instead of running being something I had to do, it became something I wanted to do because I could. *Run because you can* became my mantra, along with *Run for those who can't*. I ran several times a week. Anytime I looked out the window and saw the weather was good, I wanted to hit the trail. I devised multiple routes of varying lengths and terrains. I started running longer distances: five-, six-, seven-, and eight-mile runs.

Upon my initial cancer diagnosis, I downloaded a fitness application to my phone to track and record the number of miles I ran, routes taken, my speed, weather conditions, and more. The app set goals for distance and time. It functioned as my own fitness coach, even talking to me in an artificial intelligence voice: *Speed up* (that one, I heard a lot). *Slow down. You're looking great. How are you feeling? Smile if you can.* And my favorite: *Enjoy being active and fit.* The application also gave me awards, badges for my fastest pace, longest run, distance targets reached, and other accomplishments. A year later, my fitness application awarded me a badge for having completed the equivalent of fourteen marathons.

For me, running came to symbolize, having the strength to live. I can handle cancer. I can survive, and I can thrive. I can be a pastor. I can preach, care for my flock, lead, and do all that's required. I can love my wife and kids. I can be there for them and give them what's needed. I can be a good friend. I can do many things I've been avoiding. I felt like *The Little Engine That Could*, continuing to chug along, and building momentum—"I think I can. I think I can. I think I can!"[5]

The self-discoveries I made running spilled over into all the other areas of my life. I can do this. I should do this because I can do this. Run because I can. Take Amy out to dinner because I can. Go to work because I can. Go to the finance committee meeting because I can. Go on the weekend getaway with your friends because you can.

A few weeks into my cancer journey, after one Sunday worship service, as I was on my way out of the sanctuary, Deb, a beloved and passionate member of my congregation, came barreling in and made a beeline towards me. She maneuvered through the outbound crowd. From the look of amazement on her face, I knew she had something to tell me.

As she closed in, I noticed the two women at her side, in tow. I wondered, *What happened. Am I in trouble? Did I say something wrong?* I hoped they came bearing good news.

Deb put her hands on my shoulders, looked me in the eyes, drew a deep breath, and unleashed a flurry of words. "Man, oh, man, I have just got to tell you, David, that was an unbelievably powerful sermon!" The ladies with her nodded as she continued. "Your preaching is really connecting with people." All three smiled gladly and warmly. "People are coming to faith in Jesus. God is using you to unleash a revival in this place. Your ministry is touching people. God is taking you to a new level. God has supercharged your ministry!"

Once Deb said it and others affirmed it, I could see it. God had been using the cancer to make me stronger, empowering my ministry and my life.

Already God had used every appointment, test, procedure, report, the waiting and uncertainty, dealing with the finances and insurance issues, and everything else to make me stronger. God had commandeered every part of my cancer experience to empower me. Cancer had forced me to step up and be strong, and more importantly, to rely on and receive God's strength. I felt confident that God would continue to use my cancer experience to make me stronger.

As the coming months unfolded, I helped the church clarify its vision and rally together. I worked with the church's leaders to guide the congregation through severe conflicts, changes, and transitions. I led challenging conversations. I provided pastoral care through some heartbreaking situations. I even conducted a funeral for a member not much older than me, who died four weeks after being diagnosed with stage four lung cancer. I worried less about what others thought, and my skin got even thicker.

Six weeks had passed since the X-ray revealed a golfball-sized mass in my lung. My oncologist finally had the biopsy results. We needed to talk about the next steps. I mustered all the faith I could, and Amy and I went to meet him.

We took a seat in the exam room, and a moment later, Dr. Crawford joined us. He wore a white coat and a friendly smile and held in his hand several sheets of paper. We had talked by phone multiple times over the last several weeks, but this was the first face-to-face appointment. A member of my church had referred him to me as "the best" and "world-renowned." I liked him a lot.

Dr. Crawford sat and explained the cancer. It was non-small cell squamous carcinoma, which is preferable to small cell because it doesn't spread as fast. A non-small cell type of lung cancer is more common among non-smokers. It did not appear to have spread to my brain. Unfortunately, it had spread (metastasized) to my sternum, lower spine, adrenal glands, and collar bone. That made it stage four, the highest and most dangerous level.

The pathology studies revealed that my lung cancer tested positive for a genetic marker/mutation known as ALK. This was good news because, in recent years, scientists had learned enough about ALK to develop targeted, effective chemotherapy medications. They could put the brakes on the renegade proteins creating the cancer cells. Less than 5 percent of people with lung cancer are "ALKies."

"If you have lung cancer," Dr. Crawford said, "this is what you want."

My chemotherapy would consist of four tablets a day. I would take the medication for the foreseeable future, maybe the rest of my life.

I should see noticeable improvement within just a few days. My coughing should soon subside, along with the pain in my side. Fatigue would be the most likely side effect. He encouraged me to keep exercising to combat fatigue.

The medication was about $15,000 a month. Despite the high cost, which shocked me, he felt confident that my insurance company would approve it.

As our visit concluded, I asked how long he thought I should expect to be alive. I never thought I would be asking and wasn't sure I wanted the answer, but stage four sounded dire, with death imminent.

Dr. Crawford replied, "Because the medication is so new as a first-line treatment, we can't know for sure. Plus, if this medication doesn't work, other treatment options exist. And with time, more treatments will likely be developed. Expect to be around for *years*."

With that, he patted me on the shoulder, smiled, said goodbye, and went on to see his next patient. I thanked him, squeezed Amy's hand, and prayed God would continue to give me strength.

Faith

The night after being told I should plan to be around for years, around two o'clock in the morning, a series of terrible visions jolted me out of deep sleep.

I could see myself hunched over the side of the bed, vomiting into a bucket, emaciated, bald, and pale. I heard the doctors explaining apologetically to Amy and my family that the treatments were ineffective. The cancer continued to spread like wildfire. "Surgery's not an option," the doctor said. "There's nothing else we can do." I watched the insurance executives decide not to pay for my chemotherapy and drop me from the plan. I watched Amy and our kids crying as we said goodbye, and then I took my last breath. I saw one of my favorite pastors presiding over my funeral, Amy shuffling through a stack of bills and paperwork, and my empty seat at my children's graduations and weddings.

It felt like the scene in *It's a Wonderful Life*, one of my favorite movies, when the angel, Clarence, showed George Bailey what the lives of those he loved would be like without him. I didn't see Clarence or anyone else, but it felt like someone had led me into my future to see the worst outcomes...just how bad cancer would be.

I tossed and turned as the onslaught of images continued throughout the night. I couldn't reach out to Amy even though she was right beside me. What would I say? I didn't want to tell her any of this. Instead, I curled up into the fetal position, fighting back tears, and waited for dawn.

In the morning, I acted like everything was normal, even though my dark night of the soul had left me shaken and exhausted. After everyone left the house, I sat in the chair beside my bed for my morning devotional time. The steaming cup of coffee in my hands comforted my achy body. I felt like I had been spiritually assaulted in the night. *Lord, what happened last night? Where were you?*

I picked up my Bible and started reading from where I had left off the day before, in the third chapter of John. "I have spoken to you of earthly things, and you do not believe; how then will you believe if I speak of heavenly things?" (John 3:12). The whole section was about believing.

Nicodemus was among those addressed. He was a very religious guy like me, a leader and teacher of the community of faith, but he didn't believe Jesus' message. "For God so loved the world that he gave his one and only Son, that whoever believes in him shall not perish but have eternal life" (John 3:16). Jesus continued to drive home the importance of believing in him and his message, and Nicodemus struggled to believe.

In the next section of my reading, Jesus meets a Samaritan woman. She is not Jewish and maybe not religious at all. Yet she believes in Jesus within a matter of minutes. I could see the bitter irony and myself in Nicodemus.

As I reflected, I could hear the Lord asking me: *Do you believe in me? Do you believe I can and will heal you? Do you believe I can make all things work together for good for you? Do you believe I can use this disease for my glory? Do you believe when you die, you will go to heaven and live with me forever? Do you really believe?*

The questions surprised me. Faith had always been part of my life. I had always believed. My mom and dad raised my brothers and me in the church. We were there every week. When I graduated high school, my youth pastor presented me with a study Bible and a copy of Oswald Chambers's *My Utmost for his Highest.* I took them both with me to college, even though I never opened either until years later.

A few months after graduating from college, my first serious relationship and first job fell apart. I crawled back to the church I grew up in, reluctantly seeking counsel from Pastor Rick. Deep down, I knew I needed God. Pastor Rick listened to me, prayed for me, and helped me experience Jesus Christ's love, forgiveness, and peace in a way I'll never forget.

A couple of years later, I joined a United Methodist Church, the one where Amy and I would be married. I started going to worship regularly. Soon after, I started teaching a Sunday school class, attending a Bible study taught by my pastor, and helping in worship. As I shared in chapter one, in my midtwenties, shortly after our first child's birth, I accepted God's call to be a pastor. I left my job in my dad's business and went to seminary. Four years later, I was ordained and appointed to serve my first church as a pastor. That was twenty years ago. *Do I believe in you? Really?*

I wanted to answer Jesus with steel-like determination. *Yes, Lord, you know I do. You know, I believe in you.* I felt like I should have been able to, but I couldn't. It wasn't that I didn't believe, but something held me back. My faith had never been tested like this. It felt inadequate. I worried that it might not be a mature enough faith to handle cancer.

Being diagnosed with cancer put my faith to the test in a way nothing else had. Never had I faced the possibility of my imminent death. I had never faced adversity that demanded so much faith.

I felt like Peter being called by Jesus to step out of the boat and onto the stormy sea to walk with Jesus on the water. If I kept my eyes on Jesus, I could walk on water. I could handle cancer. But like Peter, the stormy waters commanded my attention and caused me to take my eyes off Jesus. The moment I looked away from Jesus, I started to sink into a sea of doubt. On more than one occasion, I could feel Jesus reaching out to catch me and hear him saying, "You of little faith, why did you doubt?" (Matthew 14:31).

The challenging circumstances revealed some of my faith faults. "Holy amnesia": I would forget everything God had already done for me and all God's promises. "Peekaboo faith": I believe you if I can see you, God. And my personal favorite, "Stinking Thinking": Instead of thinking positively about what can happen with God for whom "nothing is impossible" (Luke 1:37, ESV), I would start thinking that everything was somehow impossible. No one wants to be around you when you're "stinking thinking." I didn't want to be around me.

I recalled an assignment from one of my favorite seminary professors, Dr. Davis. We were studying the great pastor, poet, and mystic John Donne. Dr. Davis asked us to pick one of his sermons and show how it could be applicable today. I spent several days writing a long paper about how it wasn't possible. A few days later, I got my paper back with a big, fat, red "F" written on the front, along with a note from Dr. Davis, reminding me that the assignment was to imagine how the sermon *could* be used today. Fortunately, for my GPA, she allowed me a chance to try again.

I accepted her offer and rewrote the essay and rewrote one of Donne's sermons, "The Fear of the Lord, " which I have since preached multiple times. It's made a big difference in the lives of many people, including myself.

I will never forget that lesson. It wasn't just about academia. It was also about me and my faith. I spent way too much time envisioning, sometimes in grand scale and meticulous detail, how things were not possible, how badly it would all fall apart. That's what my night of terrible visions was about. In the same way, I needed to approach my cancer with faith in what God could do and all the good things possible.

I knew the difference that faith makes and how important it is. Faith has the power to change our lives and the world. I remembered Jesus' bold promise of the power of faith.

"Truly I tell you, if you have faith as small as a mustard seed, you can say to this mountain, 'Move from here to there,' and it will move. Nothing will be impossible for you" (Matthew 17:20).

I preached and taught on Jesus' mind-blowing promise countless times. Faith in Jesus can move the mountain. With just a little faith, even if the mountain doesn't move right now, Jesus can move it or take you over its top. At the very least, faith will change your perception of the mountain. It won't look as insurmountable. God will show you the way over it, around it, or through it. Or Jesus will simply throw it into the sea.

Without faith, you're left with an immovable mountain staring you in the face, taunting and sneering, and casting its shadow over you. Without faith, you are left with only fear. Faith and fear are like day and night—it's one or the other.

What you believe determines what you think, expect, see, and usually get. We encourage our children saying, *You have to believe it to achieve it. Visualize success.* If I expect my day to be terrible, it probably will be. If I expect the day to be great, chances are it will be. If I look for them, I'll find the goodness and blessings of God waiting for me.

While cancer showed many of the shortcomings of my faith, I expected that God would also use cancer to help me stand taller in my faith.

At Sunday worship, a few days after my night of stinking thinking, about a dozen young children came to the front of the worship space, with their leaders. The leaders explained that the children wanted to knight me and present me with the "the armor of God" so I would be prepared for my cancer battle.

I came as summoned and took my place among them. One of the younger boys, a little guy with a little voice, read: "Sir David, by order of the King, we are here to present you with the full armor of God so that you can be successful in all your battles. Please kneel."

As I did, one of the older girls took the microphone and began reading the Bible verse: "Put on the full armor of God so that you can take your stand" (Ephesians 6:11).

As she read, the children took turns presenting the armor. Two giggling boys wrapped the "belt of truth" around my waste. It had been convincingly made of silver duct tape and had

BELT OF TRUTH printed in large black letters across the front. As they attempted to fasten it in place, I admired their handy work. Then one of the boys blurted, "It's too small! We can't get it on." The congregation erupted in laughter, and I tried to suck in my belly.

Next, two of the girls presented the "breastplate of salvation," a t-shirt featuring a large white ribbon on the front, representing the fight against lung cancer, and an encouraging Bible verse. On one side, the children had written their names as best they could. On the other side, they had written Bible verses ("John 3:16" and others). They insisted I immediately put it on over my shirt. Of course, it was two sizes too small.

Two children presented the "Gospel shoes," a pair of Carolina blue booties like the kind surgeons wear over their shoes. They lifted my feet and slid them on over my shoes. I started to lose my balance and almost fell, but some of the children pushed me back upright.

They presented an orange wig for the "helmet of salvation" and a hand-crafted "sword of the spirit." One of the boys whispered, in my ear, "Be careful. The handle falls off easy." They draped a cape, which is not scriptural, over my shoulders, and finally presented me with the "shield of faith."

I thanked the children, and to their delight, triumphantly hoisted up the shield of faith. The children and the congregation erupted with cheering, clapping, and shouts of victory. I felt like Mel Gibson in the movie *Braveheart*.

As I held up the shield, I saw the children's names written on the back, in their handwriting: Madeline, Kathryn, Ryan, Cooper, and others. Some had added pictures, smiley faces, and hearts. Tears flooded my eyes.

The children's gift ministered to me. It was as if they had somehow known exactly what I needed. As they say, "And a little child shall lead them."

After my diagnosis, I intentionally tried to do things that encouraged my faith. I made a "faith" playlist of my favorite songs about faith and listened to them throughout the day. I looked more often at the pictures on the walls of our home that communicated messages of faith. I allowed myself more time for my daily devotions—the time I spent alone reading the Bible, reflecting, journaling, praying, and drinking coffee.

The Bible has always been central to my faith. Reading Scripture has helped me find, sustain, grow, and keep my faith for many years. The Bible speaks often about faith. As a Methodist, I believe Scripture contains everything necessary for our salvation. Throughout my life, God's Word has given me strength and guidance, reminded me of God's promises, and made me aware of God's presence.

Many Bible verses and stories impacted my faith during the early days and weeks of living with cancer, but two changed everything. The first was John 11:4: "This sickness will not end in death. No, it is for God's glory so that God's Son may be glorified through it."

A few days after my dark night of the soul, in my morning devotional time, a second Bible verse rocked my world. I was reading the story of Jesus and his disciples encountering a man who had been blind since birth (John 9). "Rabbi," his disciples said to him, "why was this man born blind? Was it because of his own sins or his parents' sins?" (John 9:2, NLT). Their reason for asking, we do not know. Maybe they felt injustice or sympathy for the man.

Whatever the case, they asked the question we all ask when bad things happen—Why? Why lung cancer? Why me? We spend a lot of time looking for explanations and reasons when bad things happen.

I listened to Jesus' answer to the disciples' question: "Neither this man nor his parents sinned, but this happened so that the works of God might be displayed in him" (John 9:3).

It couldn't have been any clearer. Again, it seemed that Jesus spoke these words to me. *David, cancer happened so that people can see God working in your life!*

At that moment, it was as if the scales fell from my eyes. My mind filled with many works of God related to my cancer.

I was awestruck and astonished by the ways God had worked in response to my cancer even before I knew I had cancer. Just a few months before my diagnosis, Amy was forced to repeat a semester of nursing school. During her extra, unneeded, and unwanted clinical education assignment, the school assigned her to work daily, for several weeks, on the hospital's pulmonary unit. During that time, she heard patients coughing in ways that sounded eerily familiar. Recognizing the possible danger that I might be in, she insisted I see my doctor. She was, of course, right. The doctors found the golf-ball-sized tumor in my right lung. Without Amy and that blessed semester, I might not be alive.

Just fourteen months before cancer showed up, a disappointing ending to an otherwise phenomenal ministry assignment forced a challenging move. The way the church decided to have me go, the timing—moving the summer before Marcie's senior year, having to sell our house with little time— none of it made sense. It would be a step up for me vocationally and a better commute for Amy. Still, the move disrupted our kids' lives and seemed wrong. After the cancer diagnosis, our unwanted move proved to be providential, and just what we needed. Our new home sat only eight miles from the world-renowned Duke Cancer Clinic.

One of the parishioners at my new church worked at Duke University Hospital and reached out to me. He had heard of the discovery of the tumor in my lung. I had no idea whom to see. He connected me with an excellent thoracic surgeon and a radiation oncologist. Miraculously, both saw me right away. I was even more amazed to find out Dr. Crawford was one of the leading thoracic oncologists in the world.

As I thought of these and other works of God's power, I recalled one of my favorite Bible verses: "All things work together for good for those who love God and are called according to his purposes" (Romans 8:28). Never had this truth been more self-evident.

I could see God's mighty works in the weeks since the cancer diagnosis and in this present moment. I had faced cancer's fears and grown in courage. I had faced my workaholism and taken steps towards genuinely living in grace. I had come face to face with my anger and unforgiveness and begun to move towards forgiveness and peace. Instead of giving up in the face of cancer, I had gotten my get-up-and-go. *Carpe Diem!* I had become a better husband and dad. My ministry had been energized. My relationship with God felt more intimate.

I could see God working in my future. I knew much more remained to be done in me, and I felt excited about it all. I could also visualize Jesus healing me. I remembered the words, "This sickness will not end in death," and I still believed. Curing me of cancer would be the mightiest work of God. I could see the day when Dr. Crawford would tell me, "The cancer is gone."

I don't think I've ever had a devotional moment like that since. Articulating the profound impact of this singular verse— "This happened so that the works of God might be displayed in him" (John 9:3)—on my life severely challenges my vocabulary. Understanding cancer as an opportunity for God to show off his mighty power in my life changed the experience entirely and grew my faith by leaps and bounds.

After that, more than ever, I could see God's mighty works every day, in almost everything. Whatever miracles God had already worked in my past, God could do now. I think you generally see what you expect to see. You go looking for trouble, and you find it. You look for reasons to give up, you find them. I went looking for God, and I found him.

You might say I put on a pair of "faith glasses," a corrective prescription pair designed to help me better see God's works. With them on, I could see God working in every dimension of my life. Without them, life became blurry and confusing.

It wasn't just sightseeing. God seemed to let me be a part of the action. By faith, I was making things happen. Jesus said, "Ask, and it will be given to you; seek, and you will find; knock, and the door will be opened to you" (Mathew 7:7). That's an invitation to faith. Well, I was asking, knocking, and looking, and things were happening. I was receiving and finding all I needed and more. Doors and hearts were opening in ways that often blew my mind. All of this caused my faith to grow exponentially.

It may sound Pollyannaish or make-believe, but it was true for me. I started to worry less about having too much faith and more about the times I didn't have enough. I wondered how often I hadn't experienced or seen God's mighty work because I didn't have enough faith. I didn't want to make that mistake again.

The day of my "works of God" revelation, near bedtime, my son Caleb, twelve years old at the time, came into my room and sat beside me on the bed. With a concerned look on his face, he cautiously said, "Dad, what's the worst thing that could happen?"

I thought about my night of terrible visions and shuddered. I thought about my meeting with Doctor Crawford— "Expect to be around for years." I also thought of all I had learned about faith.

I put my arm around Caleb, held him tight, and reassured him, "Caleb, we don't need to think about the worst that can happen. We believe that God loves us. We believe that God is with us. We believe God can do all things. We believe that God can heal me. And we believe in heaven. Do you believe that?"

"Yes," he replied confidently.

"Great! Let's think about God healing your dad. Let's think about all the best things that can happen. Let's pray and ask God for the best things. Okay, Caleb?"

"Okay, Dad." His countenance changed in a flash, and he smiled a big smile. His natural energy returned to his body. He hugged me, and said, "I love you, Dad," then zipped out of my room and onto something else.

"I love you, too, Caleb!" I shouted after him.

A little while later, I went to tell him goodnight. I could hear him playing his guitar and singing. I stopped at his closed door, and with gratitude and joy, listened to him sing about the "God of Miracles" and how we believe in Jesus and his healing power. *Go, Caleb!*

Three months later, I went to the cancer clinic for my first follow-up appointment with Dr. Crawford, my oncologist, since starting chemotherapy.

As Amy and I headed over, I felt good and optimistic. I had tolerated the chemotherapy amazingly well. The pain in my side and the coughing had gone away within a few days, as the doctor had hoped. The only side effects had been the occasional mild fatigue.

I told my friends and family I believed the healing was already happening. The cancer might even be gone. I had every reason to expect the results of the CT scan of my lungs to be good. I felt full of faith in Jesus.

After the routine bloodwork and the CT scan and a long wait in the lobby, we were finally in the examination room. As I sat in the observation chair and waited, I remembered Jacob's struggle. I breathed deep and prayed, "God, I will not let you go until you bless me. Amen." I prayed at least one of those blessings would be a good report.

My oncologist knocked and came into the room with a fist full of papers and wearing his usual attire and a smile.

He sat on the stool and rolled over to me with a few sheets of paper in one hand, and patted me on my knee with the other. With a happy expression, he pulled out one with a black and white image of my lungs on it.

"David, these are remarkable results. They're even better than we had hoped to see. The tumor in your lung has shrunk by more than fifty percent. In addition, we can see evidence of healing in the surrounding areas to which the cancer had spread. Congratulations."

He was pleased. I was absolutely elated. In just three months, the cancer was half-way gone. Thank you, Jesus! I would continue the treatments, and he would see me in another three months.

I left feeling blessed, amazed, and grateful. Never had my faith been so confirmed, and never had I been so full of faith in Jesus.

Provision

The questions jolted me awake at two o'clock in the morning. Is our life insurance policy up to date? When does it expire? Have we been making the payments on time? Did we set it up correctly? Is it enough? Where is the paperwork? Whether I had been dreaming about it or thinking about it, subconsciously, my heart raced.

Cancer conjured up a storm of fears. Financial fears topped the list: PET scans, CT scans, MRIs, biopsies, chemotherapy, doctors' appointments—cancer care could cost tens of thousands, hundreds of thousands, or even millions of dollars. We had been limping along for so long financially that we had no room for any extra expenses. Our youngest had recently broken his pinky finger, and those additional expenses challenged us.

As I lay in bed, clenching my fists, I declared to myself, *If I die, I want to be confident, if I do nothing else, that I leave my family better off financially*. It sickened me to think of dying and leaving them in even worse shape.

For the next two hours, I tossed and turned and searched my mind for answers about the life insurance policy. None came only more questions. Finally, my anxiety forced me out of bed, and I headed downstairs to our office where we keep our important papers.

I flipped through every folder in our filing cabinets. Checked every desk drawer, swept each bookshelf, looking above, below, and behind, and found nothing. I checked drawers and cabinets in the other rooms. Still no luck. I came back to the office and started pulling files out of the cabinets and dropping each onto the floor. I would have screamed if everyone hadn't still been sleeping.

A little after six, the sun came up, followed by Amy and the kids as they prepared for work and school. Passing by the office on the way to the kitchen, each one looked and saw me sitting on the floor, in the middle of a splattering of files and papers. All the drawers were opened. It looked like a white-collar crime scene. With a forced smile and a thumbs-up, I assured them everything was okay.

As soon as they left the house, I phoned our insurance company. Not wanting to elicit concern, I took a deep breath and then calmly told our agent I would like to check the status of our policy, ensure it's up to date, and review the benefits. I then requested that he mail me a summary for my files, which seemed to be in slight disarray.

After a brief hold, the agent confirmed the policy to be up to date. In his opinion, we had set up the policy correctly, the same way he'd set up his own, which reassured me. He explained that our policy is a thirty-year term policy that will end on October 15, 2029, shortly after our youngest child would likely graduate from college. If I died before that day, the policy would pay a $1 million benefit. This was the most affordable way to make sure the kids and Amy were taken care of if I died.

Somehow remaining calm, I thanked the agent, said goodbye, and hung up. I jumped up and pumped my fist in the air. "Yes! Yes! Yes!" I kicked some files across the floor, danced for joy, and thanked God.

As I happy-danced around my office, the somber significance of October 15, 2029, came into focus and ended my elation. If I died before then, my family would get a million dollars. Just like that, all their financial needs would be taken care of—college, house, car, debt. They would have more money than they had ever had in their lives. But if I lived a minute longer, if I were still around on October 16th, they wouldn't get anything. The realization took the wind out of me.

That morning, standing in my office, I heard God asking, *Which is most important to you? Being with your family or giving them a million dollars? If your family had to choose between you and the money, what do you think they would want most?* I smiled as I imagined my kids saying, "Sorry, Dad, we love you, but we need the cash!" I knew the answer beyond a shadow of a doubt. They would choose me, and I would choose them.

God seemed to be asking me a more profound question. Do you trust me to provide for your financial needs? Do you trust me to provide for your family?

The Bible tells us that God faithfully provides. Jehovah, one of the names of God, found in the Bible, means "the Lord will provide" (Genesis 22:14). God, our creator, provides life and everything needed to sustain it. The Lord provided for Israel, his special people—manna, bread from heaven, water from a rock, a pillar of fire to lead them by night, a cloud to give them shade and lead them by day, and clothes and sandals that never wore out. The Lord will provide for us.

I love the Psalmist's interpretation of God as the provider: "All creatures look to you to give them their food at the proper time. When you give it to them, they gather it up; when you open your hand, they are satisfied with good things" (Psalm 104:27-28).

God gave us the greatest gift possible, Jesus. Jesus provided what people needed: food for five thousand, wine for the wedding party, healing for the hurting, teaching for the clueless, friendship for the lonely, and purpose for his disciples. He taught those who would listen to trust God's provision. He taught us to pray—"give us this day our daily bread" (Matthew 6:11). Most importantly, Jesus gave his life for us on the cross so we could all be saved.

Paul points out the obvious. "he who did not spare his own Son, but gave him up for us all—how will he not also, along with him, graciously give us all things?" (Romans 8:32). The bottom line: God will provide.

As a lifelong practicing Christian, going to church my whole life and having lead churches for twenty years, 1 knew all of this. 1 must have prayed thousands of times the Lord's Prayer, with its petition for "daily bread." 1 had led stewardship campaigns teaching people to give and to trust that God would provide.

A little later that morning, in my devotional time, 1 continued to thank God that our life insurance was in order. As 1 prayed, 1 heard Jesus' words:

> Do not worry about your life, what you will eat or drink; or about your body, what you will wear. Look at the birds of the air...And why do you worry about clothes? See how the flowers of the field grow.... Seek first his kingdom and his righteousness, and all these things will be given to you as well.
>
> —(Matthew 6:25-34).

God had always been faithful to me. 1 could write a book about the amazing ways God has provided for me financially— big and small.

About ten years earlier, my car broke down. It needed expensive repairs 1 couldn't afford. Having no choice but to fix my car, 1 took it to the shop. 1 told the front desk manager, Rock, to go easy on me. Later that day, he called and said it was ready.

1 went back to the shop with trepidation. 1 was afraid to ask about the cost. 1 hoped the total would be something 1 could squeeze onto my credit card. When 1 walked into the office, Rock called me over to him. He slid the invoice across the counter, along with my keys.

"You're all set," he said.

"What do 1 owe you?" 1 sheepishly said as 1 scanned the bill for the price, unable to find anything.

At the bottom, he had written, *N/C*.

"What does N/C mean?" I said. "I hope it doesn't mean non-computable." I gave a nervous laugh.

"No," Rock said, with a smile on his face, "that means no charge. The Lord told me to provide this repair to you free of charge."

Almost every year, someone offered a vacation home to us for a week. For our summer vacation in 2018, our first since my cancer diagnosis, we stayed at Holden Beach in North Carolina, in the biggest and most beautiful house we had ever stayed in, and it was oceanfront. Because it was big enough for us to bring family and friends, we had an especially great time. During the day, we stayed on the beach, and walked easily to the house for food, drinks, and other necessities, whenever we liked. At night, we sat in the rocking chairs on the porch, listening to the ocean, feeling the breeze, and looking at the stars. We enjoyed cooking meals in the home's enormous kitchen and eating together at a table for twelve. We played games and put together puzzles. Amy and I slept in the master bedroom in a luxurious bed with an unobstructed view of the ocean. We had a grand time.

A couple of months earlier, we weren't sure we would be able to afford a vacation. A week in that beach house at primetime would have cost several thousand dollars. It belonged to Julie, Terry's sister, whom I mentioned in chapter four, and her husband. They gave us the time as a gift. Julie wouldn't even allow us to pay the usual cleaning charge. Talk about provision.

When we were preparing to move to Chapel Hill, one of the members whom I had not yet met, called me. He suggested it would be good for our family to take a special trip before starting my new assignment. He understood the transition hadn't been an easy one. If we'd had all our passports, he would have sent us to Europe. Knowing we had three kids, he suggested we spend a week at Disney World. He insisted we stay in the Grand Floridian, inside the park, which would allow us the convenience of taking the monorail into the parks from our hotel. He also wanted us to have a generous meal plan so we wouldn't have to worry about any food. He asked me to call, figure out the details, and then let him know the cost. I hesitated to let him know the trip's final price tag. Without hesitation, he paid for the trip and even instructed the hotel to keep his credit card on file for our incidentals. To date, this remains the most special family vacation we have ever had. It was magical.

God had provided in many other ways. I remember one friend, after sensing our need, gave me a handful of cash out of the blue. On one occasion, when we sold a home, the real estate agent who sold our house refused to take a commission. An orthodontist from one of our churches provided our oldest daughter's braces for free. One of my best friends gave me his old car when mine was on its last legs. We have received generous love offerings from each church we've served, upon our leaving.

Time and time again, God had provided for our needs in the most amazing ways. God had always been faithful. I had no reason to believe God wouldn't continue to provide. Despite all this, as I considered the costs of cancer, I struggled to remember and rely on God's faithful provision.

Before cancer showed up, my financial challenges were already beyond my control. A few years earlier, Amy had gone back to school to become a nurse and fulfill her life's calling, and my calling never seemed to pay enough. I was committed to her success. I knew it would take time and money, but I had underestimated how much of both. It took longer than we expected. A year from her projected graduation, we were barely hanging on—pinching pennies, cycling through cards, and accumulating debt. Financial relief wouldn't come until she graduated.

Despite the reality of our situation, I continued to try to make our finances work. I worried and agonized, stressed, and doubted, budgeted, and forecasted the bad things that would happen. I spent hours balancing our books and trying to be in control. I would become angry and raise my voice. I tried everything, but nothing changed.

Now, with cancer and its anticipated financial costs, I had to acknowledge things were officially beyond my control. I had no choice but to trust God to provide. I considered the possibility that God had woken me that morning to teach me a lesson. I sensed God would use cancer to cure me of my fears of not having enough and grow my trust in his provision.

In the Old Testament's story of the Israelites' exodus, the people have escaped Egypt. They are fleeing through the desert to the Promised Land, with Pharaoh's army in hot pursuit. They come to the Red Sea. They can't cross it or go back. Pharaoh's army has them trapped. It's either face the sword or swim. With their backs against the wall, they surely wonder why on earth, God had brought them there.

Interestingly, the Scripture reveals that God lead them to that place, knowing full well they'd get stuck there. Otherwise, they would have already given up and returned to their Egyptian bondage. More importantly, God put them there so they could learn to trust God to provide a way out. They had to trust God to make a way. God showed up in a big way, parting the sea before their eyes. They walked through the sea, experiencing the miracle of God's provision firsthand, but only coming from a place of helplessness.

Similarly, our financial challenges had us in a bind. Surrounded by overwhelming financial hardship, I had no choice but to trust God to provide the financial resources we needed to live and deal with cancer's costs, whatever they might be.

One day, a representative from the hospital's billing department called to review the financial cost of the bronchoscopy—the surgical biopsy with the camera and special equipment going down my throat and into my lungs. The representative started telling me how much it cost, how much my health insurance would pay, and how much I would have to pay. With pen and paper in hand, I prepared to write down the information.

She said the total cost was $18,000. I marveled at how an outpatient procedure that took less than a couple of hours could cost so much. As I wrote the number, I heard the representative say, "How would you like to pay for that, Mr. Gira? Debit or credit?"

"Credit or debit?" I don't think that's what she said, but that's what I heard. The pencil fell from my hand, and I leaned back in my chair. "Pardon me. Please repeat that?"

"Mr. Gira, your portion is $1,800. How would you like to pay for that?"

After a moment of awkward silence, waiting for me to respond, she continued, "Mr. Gira, you can pay a lesser amount if you need to, and we can work out a payment arrangement."

I could hear my mother-in-law, Dot: "Pay them a dollar, Bob." We already had too many monthly payments. Amy had prepped me for this. "Tell them you don't want to pay until after the insurance has processed the claim and paid its portion."

I doubted that approach would work, and I didn't have the guts to ask, but I really couldn't pay anything. On my computer, I checked our bank account's balance. Timidly, I said, "Can I pay fifty dollars today?"

The representative didn't seem excited about my offer. But after a brief pause, she agreed that would work just fine.

After finishing the call, I frightfully imagined the cost of scans, procedures, medications, and everything else that lay ahead. I could see the payment plan becoming like a house payment. I'm surprised I didn't hyperventilate and pass out onto the floor.

Later that same day, I received a short, unexpected text message from a man from my church. To honor his desire to remain anonymous, I will call him Philip. He asked if I would like to meet him for a meal the next day. He had been following my health crisis and expressed concern for my family and me. I welcomed the opportunity.

We met the next day at a local restaurant. After we talked about our families, work, and church, Philip asked me about my cancer journey. He expressed interest in the cost of my health care, my insurance benefits, and details regarding my out-of-pocket expenses. I acknowledged my concerns regarding the mounting cost of my medical care and shared with him my call experience regarding the billing for the bronchoscopy.

As breakfast concluded and we prepared to part ways, Philip asked me to give him the medical bills I had received for the previous scans and appointments at my earliest convenience. With a whimsical, mischievous smile, he said, "I may be able to help with that."

Despite some of my reservations about receiving such generous help from someone I had known only a year, I trusted this to be God's hand at work providing for me. No other explanation sufficed. The next day, I took Philip the few bills I had received, which amounted to about $2,000, and dropped them off at his house.

Two hours later, I received a text from Philip saying; *I have put the checks in the mail. When you get your next bill, please give that to me also. Thanks!*

Amazed by his generosity, I thanked him and thanked God. I couldn't believe this was happening. At the same time, I couldn't believe that I hadn't believed God would provide in some way like this. I knew God worked that way. He always had and always would.

Over the next twelve months, Philip texted me every couple of weeks, inviting me to a meal and asking if I had any "paperwork." We met several times, and have continued to meet to this day.

In addition to financially supporting me through my cancer journey, Philip has blessed our family in many beautiful ways. His generosity has enabled us to do things and go places that would not otherwise have been possible. In addition to financial support, he has provided each one of us with individualized attention, wisdom, and encouragement.

"Philip" refers to the early Christian church at Philippi. Paul wrote a famous letter to the Philippian church, which is one of the books found in the Bible and known as Philippians. In it, Paul repeatedly thanked the members of that community of

Christians for their financial support of him and his missionary work.

"I thank my God in all my remembrance of you, always in every prayer of mine for you all making my prayer with joy, because of your partnership in the gospel from the first day until now" (Philippians 1:3-5, ESV).

Throughout the book of Philippians, Paul thanks his faithful supporters. They have been his partners. Similarly, my friend Philip often referred to his support of me as a "partnership." I believe he felt called by God to be my partner in my cancer journey by providing the financial resources needed.

I thanked God for Philip. Over and over, I joined with Paul in saying, "I thank my God every time I remember you" (Philippians 1:3). Philip's generosity helped me overcome my fears about the cost of cancer care. He took away a significant cause for concern. More importantly, he witnessed to and taught me about God's faithful provision.

My newfound confidence transformed my experiences of checking in for medical appointments and procedures. Instead of being afraid, I started to feel like Luke Skywalker from *Star Wars*, using my Jedi powers. When the receptionist asked for the payment, I replied, "You don't need a payment from me today. You will bill me." As expected, he or she responded, "Mr. Gira, we don't need a payment from you today. We will bill you." To which, I would respond, in my head, "May the Force be with you."

I also thanked God (and still do) for the blessing of having excellent health insurance. When my oncologist told me my chemotherapy would costs $15,000 a month and that I would have to take it for the foreseeable future, possibly the rest of my life, I was terrified. I did the math: $108,000 for one year, $900,000 for five years, and 2 million dollars if I lived for six years. There was some encouraging news; it turned out, I was worth twice as much alive as I was dead!

Somehow, by the grace of God and with the persuasion of Dr. Crawford, my insurance company approved the needed medication for my treatment, and it turned out to be extremely effective. Putting the icing on the cake, because I had already met my out-of-pocket maximum for the year, I didn't have to pay anything, not even a copay, for the chemotherapy for the first few months. The following year, when I did have to pay a copay, it was $5. Amazing.

I still don't understand how it's possible to receive $15,000-per-month medicine for $5. I am concerned about the high cost of medicine and the many who don't have health insurance or access to the medications and care they need. Serious reflection and changes are required. While I think of all of that, the $5 payment has served as an effective monthly reminder that God will provide.

One morning, Bible in hand, I reflected more on Paul's words: "I thank my God every time I remember you" (Philippians 1:3)." I offered a prayer of thanks to God for the generous people in my life.

As I thought about God's generous provision, I began to hear within me the names of friends, parishioners, family members, and others who had provided for my family and me. I saw the faces of parishioners who had gifted my family with places to vacation. I saw the people who had given me financial gifts. I saw my friend who gave me his car. I saw those who helped me with the financial expenses of cancer. I saw my parents, whose love had been steadfast all my life. Soon, I had written down the names of a hundred people. Memories of these and other generous people flooded my mind as my heart overflowed with gratitude.

My eyes were soaked with tears of appreciation. The Lord had shown me many of the people he had blessed me with and used to provide for my needs. I gave thanks to God for them all.

I could hear Jesus calling me to keep believing and trusting him. I could be assured that God would provide for all my needs.

Patience

At my first follow-up visit after starting chemotherapy, my doctor reported that my scan showed the tumor had shrunk by 50 percent. I was elated and overjoyed.

Three months later, it was time for my next follow-up appointment. I went with high hopes, expecting that the remaining 50 percent of the tumor would be gone. *God, I know you're able.*

I felt even better than I had three months earlier. After six months of cancer and treatments, I still had no significant side effects. I continued to live unhindered, feeling more empowered. Every dimension of my life seemed enhanced.

I could see it all in my mind's eye. My oncologist would walk into the observation room with his papers in hand, smiling broadly, throw them up in the air, and say, "The cancer's gone! You're cured." With that, his team would burst through the door with streamers, noisemakers, confetti, and a celebratory cake. I could even taste the cake.

The day of the appointment, after having blood drawn and then the scans, we waited in the observation room. Dr. Crawford entered the room, as envisioned. After a few minutes of small talk, he showed us images from the scan and told us he had great news: "The tumor has shrunk by another fifteen percent. "

Amy and my parents expressed their delight. "Great!
news."

"How Wonderful!"

"That's awesome."

Dr. Crawford continued, "The progress continues to be
remarkable, exceeding our hopes."

Amy smiled at me and squeezed my hand. My happy
parents breathed a sigh of relief.

Despite everyone's optimism, I felt a huge wave of
sadness and disappointment crash over me. I felt angry, hurt,
and crushed. The cancer had shrunk, which was great, but
it wasn't gone. As they continued talking, I tried to hide my
disappointment and pain.

I tried to joke about it. I asked my doctor for a note
excusing me from my church's finance committee meeting that
evening. Happy to play along, he wrote it on his prescription
pad, with typical barely legible physician's handwriting. While
we all got a kick out of it, I seriously wasn't ready to be around
anyone. I needed time to recover from what felt like a huge
disappointment.

Dr. Crawford, sensing my disappointment, offered some
words of reassurance.

"Healing is a process," he said, "sometimes taking months
or years. Even if today's scan had only shown that the tumor
hadn't gotten any bigger, that would have been a great report. To
have fifteen percent shrinkage is phenomenal, excellent."

With that, he stood, put his hand on my shoulder, looked
me in the eye, and said, "Try to be patient."

I had never been patient. I may not have wanted to admit
it, but my family knew it. I would try to be patient, but I couldn't
make any promises.

As a child, I couldn't wait to unwrap Christmas presents.
If the gift tantalized me too much, I might unwrap it, see what
it was, and rewrap it. As a young adult, I got myself in debt over
my head as soon as I got my first credit card. I couldn't wait to

earn money before I spent it. That tells you everything you need to know.

As an adult, my wife Amy has told me a thousand times over the twenty years we've been married: "You have no patience." I have struggled to be patient while waiting for her to finish getting ready, get off the phone, finish her TV show, come to bed, have dinner ready, answer my question, return my message, and complete her nursing degree.

Impatience runs in my family. I can remember sitting in the backseat of my grandpa's station wagon as a kid, listening to him honking the horn repeatedly to hurry up my grandma. I hate to confess it, but I have sounded my horn more than a couple times. He loved to take me fishing, but we never caught anything that I can remember, probably because we couldn't leave our hooks in the water long enough.

My kids had seen my impatience. I can see my daughter, Marcie, now getting ready for kindergarten, looking up at me over her shoulder as she tied her shoes, carefully making her precious loops while at the same time telling me, "Be patient, Daddy."

Now all grown up, my kids were still reminding me to be patient. We recently went out to dinner, and I got upset that the food was taking so long. Hannah, with her head in her hands, elbowed me and said, "Geeze, Dad, chill out. We're not the only people in the restaurant. Be patient."

I tended not to be patient enough, even with myself. My impatience enabled my perfectionism and fed my inner critic. You should have this figured out by now, moron. Why are you...? When will you...? How much longer will you...? If a friend spoke to me as I talk to me, we wouldn't stay friends.

My impatience had gotten me in trouble over the years. I often spoke too soon. I didn't listen long enough. I got my feelings hurt or lost my cool. I said something hurtful—something cold, mean, critical, insensitive. I acted too soon and made some terrible decisions because I wouldn't wait.

I recalled a recent trip to a coffee shop. I had been watching the talented barista make two masterpiece drinks for Amy and me. While we watched in awe, another customer came in and began to wait with us for his turn to be served. After a few minutes, I could feel his impatience building. While the barista carefully sprayed the whipped cream on the top of the first drink, I saw the other customer leave. A couple of minutes later, the barista slid the second drink across the bar to us. We sipped our mind-blowing delicious drinks. Our fellow would-be patron missed out on the coffee drink of a lifetime because he didn't have the patience to wait five more minutes.

The customer reminded me of myself and the importance of being patient and the blessings one often receives for waiting. I hated to know how many good and wonderful things I could have had if I could have waited a few minutes longer. I could have been there for that awesome performance my kid gave. Amy and I could have enjoyed many more special times together if I had been able to wait patiently. My plan at work would have been a big success if I had just stuck with it a little longer.

Early in my cancer journey, I realized there's a reason why a patient is called *"patient."* As I searched for a parking space at the hospital, I had to be patient, circling my way up towards the top of the parking deck. I had to be patient as I waited to see my doctor, even if he was ninety minutes behind schedule. I had to be patient as a nurse tried to start my IV for the fourth time. I had to be patient as the insurance company decided whether to approve my claim. I had to be patient and endure a second biopsy because the first didn't work, and then be patient as the pathology studies were completed so I could be placed on the most effective chemotherapy. I had to be patient as I waited for the medicine to work. I had to be patient as I waited for the next scan. And I had to be patient with the healing process, no matter how slow it seemed. Fifteen percent shrinkage in three months! I had to be patient, terminally patient. I had no choice.

I could not imagine there being anything harder to wait for than the healing of cancer. I wanted it out of my body immediately. The longer it was there, the more time it had to spread. The stakes had never been higher. Everything was a matter of life or death. I couldn't afford to wait, but I had to wait. I had to be patient.

Before cancer, I had no idea what it meant to have to be patient. All my previous experiences with patience had been like playing little league. Cancer had bumped me up to the big leagues. Now I had to be patient every day, and much more was at stake. Cancer revealed my impatience not just with the disease, but with everything and everyone.

The Bible has a lot to say about being patient. I could quote verses about patience, starting with my favorite.

"I waited patiently for the Lord. He inclined and heard my cry. He brought me up out of the pit, out of the miry clay" (Psalm 40:1).

I grew up singing those words. U2 was my favorite rock and roll band, and I loved their song "40." I realized years later that the words were from Psalm 40 in the Bible.

God is patient with us. That's the starting point. "You are merciful, LORD! You are kind and patient and always loving" (Psalm 145:8, CEV).

Consequently, the Bible tells us we should be patient with each other. "Be patient, bearing with one another in love" (Ephesians 4:2b). We all have heard, "Love is patient, love is kind" (1 Corinthians 13:4).

Unfortunately, I had never been able to practice what I preached. Perhaps God would use my cancer to cure my impatience. "With God, nothing will be impossible" (Luke 1:37, NKJV).

Two days after my follow up appointment, I shared the results of my CT scan with some staff members and Helen, one of our members who had come into the office to volunteer for the day. I confided in them my disappointment that the cancer wasn't all gone, just another 15 percent. The slowness of the progress hurt and frustrated me.

As the staff members sympathized and encouraged me. Helen leaned back in her chair, folded her arms across her chest, squinted, and scowled. Whispering, she interrupted them, "Now you listen to me. David, don't you know how fortunate you are? Imagine how many people would love to get that report. Do you think about those who won't even be alive for their next appointment? Do you know how fortunate you are to be able to wait? Wow. Shouldn't you be grateful?"

Helen's comments caught me off guard and embarrassed me. I tried not to show how much she hurt and angered me. On the outside, I listened calmly to her, but on the inside, I was yelling, *You have no idea how hard this is, how cancer has turned my life upside down, what I'm going through. Of course, I'm grateful, but I have every right to be upset. How dare you judge me.* With thinly veiled sarcasm, I thanked her and my staff, excused myself, and pulled my office door closed.

Still steaming, I sat at my desk. It didn't take long for me to acknowledge that she was right. My impatience was preventing me from being grateful for the miraculous healing I had already experienced. I was so focused on having complete healing right now that I could not be thankful for the healing already accomplished and still in process. My impatience had also made me selfish. So many others would have given everything to have gotten such a good report.

The Bible, especially the New Testament, records many accounts of stories of people receiving instantaneous healing. *Stand up and walk. Receive your sight. Come back to life. Walk out of that tomb. Be cured of your leprosy. Straighten out your crippled hand.* At times, we still see instant healing in Jesus' name. When we do, we are reminded that God is with us, still able, and willing to heal. That's what I wanted—instant healing.

In all those accounts, at first glance, each person appears to have been healed with no patience having been required. None whatsoever. But look again and consider how long each person waited for the healing moment to come. The lame man Jesus healed at the Pool of Bethesda had suffered from his infirmity for thirty-eight years (John 5:5). The woman "having an issue of blood" had been bleeding for twelve years before Jesus healed her (Luke 8:43, KJV). Lazarus had been sick for a while and then dead in the tomb for four days before Jesus restored him to life (John 11:1-44).

Everyone had to wait for healing in one way or another. Maybe all healing did require patience. Sometimes we might have to wait until the very end, perhaps even until after death.

A couple of examples from Scripture relating to patience helped me see my healing journey differently.

St. Paul suffered from a chronic ailment he referred to as the "thorn in his side." We don't know what the thorn was, but as far as we can tell from Scripture, God never removed it. Paul was never healed, even though he "pleaded" continuously to God. Instead, God replied with a promise: "My grace is sufficient for you, for my power is made perfect in weakness" (2 Corinthians 12:8).

The Lord essentially told Paul that his healing would be a life-long process. God would provide his healing through daily doses. There would be healing, but never instant, and maybe never complete. Paul needed more than a little patience. He had to be patient for the long haul.

Despite his chronic disease, Paul lived a full and fruitful life, thriving as a missionary, leader, and pastor. God used Paul's thorn and the lifelong process of healing to increase divine grace and strength in him and enable him to accomplish tremendous good for God. The thorn was a catalyst. It was a big part of his testimony. It also kept Paul humble and focused on God every moment. Christianity wouldn't be what it is now if God had given Paul instant healing.

I sensed then that God intended for my healing of cancer to be like Paul's. It would be a process and require patience. It would happen in stages. Cancer would be my thorn in my side, and I would always have it. I asked God to remove the cancer, and God did not. My thorn had gotten smaller, but it was still there. In a sense, it would always be there. With cancer, you never know if you are in remission or have been cured.

With this revelation came a decision. I could choose to be forever angry with this thorn in my side, or I could let God use it for good. I could allow it to force me to turn to and rely on God each day to sustain me. That is always the best way to position yourself. I could let God use cancer to make me more effective as a pastor and positively impact every dimension of my life. Living in the process of healing could help me grow in my relationship with God.

God gave me another *be patient* revelation shortly after Paul's. The Bible recounts in the history of the Israelites, God's chosen people, how they endure four hundred and thirty years of cruel slavery in Egypt (Exodus 12:40) before God hears their prayers and sends Moses to liberate them from Egypt. Talk about a long wait. With the help of God's miraculous signs, Moses obtains the Israelites' jailbreak. Suddenly, they are free and following Moses, their unexpected hero, through the desert, on their way to the Promised Land, a land flowing with milk and honey.

Their forty-day estimated time of arrival ended up being delayed. The forty-day trip turned into a forty-year excursion. Got patience? The Israelites hadn't gotten far before the trip revealed them to be unready and unworthy of the Promised Land. They needed more time to get to know God—time to learn to love, trust, obey, serve, worship, and enjoy God. They needed time to become the people God created them to be, people worthy of the Promise Land. Sadly, many died in the desert.

Forty years after leaving Egypt, the people are nearly ready to enter the Promised Land. God gathers them together and tells them how it's going to go down, how they'll take the land. The land he's giving them is already occupied by whole nations of people, a small point Moses failed to mention. Not to worry, however. God will send an angel ahead to drive them out before the Israelites arrive. Their enemies will run for cover when they see them coming. The land will be the Israelites'. Don't worry.

But here's what God says in the pep talk that interested me most. "But I will not drive them out in a single year, because the land would become desolate and the wild animals too numerous for you. Little by little, I will drive them out before you, until you have increased enough to take possession of the land" (Exodus 23:20-33).

In other words, they still weren't ready to have the Promised Land all at once. The land would not instantly be theirs. They would receive it gradually, day by day, year by year. The Israelites would need time to grow into the land, to become stronger and ever more faithful to God. They would have to be patient.

The Israelite's journey resonated with me. At the first follow-up visit, when the doctor said my cancer had shrunk by 50 percent, I thought God had given me a quick deliverance. I was on the fast track. I would arrive in the Promised Land in forty days. At the second follow-up visit, when he reported the cancer had shrunk by fifteen percent, it looked more like the forty-year journey. Hearing how God gave the Israelites the land "little by little" seemed to solidify that I was on the long road to healing.

Like the Israelites, I might not be ready to receive total healing right now. To be instantly 100 percent healed of disease by God would be an awesome blessing and responsibility. By God giving me healing little by little, I would have more time to become the person God wanted me to be. If God planned to use my time with cancer to make me more like Jesus, he would need more than forty years!

While it pained me to accept the slow road to healing, I found encouragement as I thought about the Israelite's amazing experiences during their forty-year trek through the desert wilderness—freedom from slavery in Egypt, the parting of the Red Sea so they could walk through on dry land, water from the rock, manna from heaven, clothes and shoes that never wore out, a cloud by day to give them shade, and a pillar of fire for the night. I could only imagine what other amazing things God might have in store for me.

At my nine-month check-in, my third quarterly follow-up visit, my doctor reported that the tumor had shrunk by another fifteen percent. The healing in the peripheral areas had also continued.

Much unlike my previous response three months earlier, I felt grateful, encouraged, and optimistic. Instead of being depressed or disheartened, I thanked God for another step in the journey of healing. I thanked God for the process. I left looking forward to the next steps of the journey.

As my one-year anniversary with cancer approached, I started thinking about having a cancer-versary party. Looking back over the past year, I felt overwhelmingly blessed by God. Every dimension of my life seemed to have been positively impacted, and my physical health had dramatically improved. I believed my one-year check-in would bring good news: continued shrinkage, maybe even cancer eliminated from my lung.

I arrived at my one-year checkup, feeling super confident. The day's agenda looked like all the preceding checkups: blood draw first, the MRI of my brain, a CT scan of the lungs, and lastly, an appointment with my oncologist to review the results.

Despite a great start to the day, the scheduled agenda went off the rails when the routine MRI took much longer than planned. Starting the standard IV took two techs and two nurses and five attempts. My veins had not shown up for the occasion. Afterward, as I suspected might happen, the oncologist's office had to reschedule my appointment so my doctor could review the scan results before seeing me.

I tried to be patient and psych myself up. *This will give me more time to be excited.* Nonetheless, I headed home feeling disappointed, with my sore arm to remind me.

The next morning, the oncologist called while I was in the middle of my staff meeting. The MRI showed cancer in my brain. I needed to come in immediately so I could meet with him and an oncology radiologist, Dr. Kelsey, and talk about the next steps.

In the office, the doctors explained their findings to me, Amy, and my parents. I appeared to have multiple tumors in my brain. All of them were small, about the size of the tip of a pencil. None were bigger than a centimeter, but there were lots of them, forty or more. He showed us the images from the scan. None of these had shown up in the MRI a year earlier. This meant the cancer had spread, metastasized, to my brain. The chemotherapy had not worked as well in my brain as it had in my lung, which now looked almost cancer-free.

As my family and I sat in disbelief and shock, Dr. Kelsey explained the next steps. I would receive eighteen "whole brain" radiation treatments. The tumors were simply too numerous to be removed one by one with targeted radiation therapy, a procedure called stereotactic radiosurgery (SRS). That meant all my healthy brain tissue would be radiated, along with the cancer.

He explained the best possible outcome and potential side effects. Radiation could effectively treat my brain's cancer so it could catch up to the good state of my lungs. I might experience nausea, fatigue, hair loss, swelling in my jaw, and potential cognitive damage. Three months after the eighteen treatments were completed, I would have another MRI to see how well I had responded and what further treatment might be needed. Hopefully, we would find that the cancer had been eliminated. If so, we would simply monitor my brain and my lungs every three months for the foreseeable future.

For a moment, I felt like crying. It felt like starting all over—lung cancer 2.0. I somehow managed to make some bad jokes about radiation to cover up my feelings. What about a head transplant? Are the tumors small because I have a little brain? Could radiation enhance my cognitive abilities? I facetiously prognosed that God might use my radiation to enhance, not diminish, my cognitive abilities. Who knows? I could end up being endowed with superpowers. I could come out of this smarter than ever. The radiation could kill the dead spots in my brain, clear the way for enhanced thinking, fire things up, uncover dormant ideas, and more.

Laughter is good medicine.

The following Tuesday, I started radiation treatments. They didn't hurt and only took a few minutes. After the first one, I had a headache, and my head felt hot, both for one day. *I am a hothead!* Dr. Kelsey said the headache was the result of my brain swelling in response to all the tumors being blasted apart. I had never been more thankful to have a headache.

After a few days, the daily radiation treatment became part of my normal routine. It disrupted my sleep schedule. I picked the earliest time slot available at 7:00 a.m. so that I could get in and out of the hospital easily and to work on time. Otherwise, my life went on normally.

As the treatments continued, I reflected on the first year of my cancer journey and looked ahead to the future. I thought about the ways God had used the cancer so far for my good—making me more courageous, more forgiving, stronger, and many other positive transformations in my life. I believed I had also become more patient. I was too afraid to ask my family if they thought so. I certainly had more work to do on the home front, but I had become more patient with God and my healing process. More cancer would give me more time to grow. If I could learn to wait patiently upon the Lord, maybe just maybe, with the Lord's help, I could learn to wait patiently upon everyone else.

Rest

My drive and determination to go and get things done exploded off the charts during the four weeks of radiation.

After each treatment, I went straight to my office. I arrived two or three hours earlier than usual, which gave me time to work on this book. I finally reached a point in my writing, where I could envision the entire book. I wrote a few of the most challenging chapters during these weeks of radiation treatments. I began organizing and editing the manuscript. I acquired contact information for potential publishers and laid out my next steps.

After the twelfth radiation treatment, I started losing my hair. That afternoon my head became increasingly itchy. Whenever I scratched my head or ran my fingers through my hair, multiple strands came out. The next morning, when I washed and rinsed my hair, I could see strands of hair on my hands, and I could feel them all over my face. A pile of hair covered the shower drain.

At work, I scratched my itchy scalp. Unable to resist, I scratched and scratched as I watched my hair fall out into my coffee cup. Hair landed across my hands, on the computer keyboard, on my shirt, and lap. My hair seemed to be everywhere.

Finding the situation unbearable, I stopped and went to the salon. I had the hairdresser give me a crew cut. She cut it down to about an eighth of an inch. Afterward, to my great pleasure, she brushed all the hair off my neck and shoulders. I felt relieved. I looked at myself in the mirror and liked the way it looked. My "new do" reminded me of my youth and maybe made me look younger. I smiled at myself in the mirror, tipped her generously, and headed back to work.

The next morning, after getting out of the shower and drying off, I saw myself in the mirror. On top of the right side of my head, the crew cut was gone. On the other side, it remained.

I found the clippers and started shaving off all the remaining hair. On his way out to school, Caleb stopped in to say goodbye just as I was attempting unsuccessfully to shave the back of my head. He looked at me, and with tenderness, asked if he could help. I surrendered the clippers, knelt in front of the bathroom counter, and he finished the job. I hugged him, told him I loved him, and he headed off to catch his school bus.

I leaned over and looked at myself in the mirror and tried to make peace with my new look. Although I know hair doesn't matter, I felt sad. I didn't like how I looked. More than that, I didn't like having my hair taken away from me. I felt robbed, defeated, and tired.

With the holiday season just around the corner, the church's calendar burst at the seams. Thanksgiving Day. The annual holiday bazaar. The Christmas open house at the parsonage. A slew of Christmas parties. End-of-year reports and staff performance reviews to complete. Staffing challenges and conflict management. Pastoral care needs, hospital and home visits, and calls to be made. And finally, all the special events, Sundays, and services of Advent and Christmas.

During it all, a flu-like illness hit me hard. I had to take off a day from work, but I went back the next day and "soldiered on." However, the illness took a real toll on me.

Each of the four Sunday services of Advent, and all three Christmas Eve services, ended the same way. As the Advent candles were lit, the congregation sang a verse of the famous hymn, "Come, Thou Long Expected Jesus."[6]

> *Come, Thou long-expected Jesus*
> *Born to set Thy people free;*
> *From our fears and sins release us,*
> *Let us find our rest in Thee.*

Week after week, I felt a growing need to find *my* rest. I began to feel more fatigued than ever. When I pushed the gas pedal, I had half my usual energy and strength. Everything seemed to take twice as much effort. Climbing the stairs was hard. Getting out of bed and getting my day going was a struggle. The occasional fatigue was becoming a daily occurrence.

All along, family, friends, colleagues, and parishioners encouraged me to take some time off from work. "Please take care of yourself."

"You look exhausted."

"You have to rest."

I thanked them for their concern, but refused to heed their advice and continued like a tired and crabby child defiantly telling his mommy and daddy, "Not tired!"

Truthfully, I resisted because I worried that if I took too much time off, my congregation and my supervisors would think less of me, lose respect for me, and my influence would diminish. We could lose all the good things that had been accomplished in the last year and a half. They might not want me back. In my twisted, workaholic mind, I had to work hard and do an excellent job for people to love me and want me. Without work, no one would love me. On top of that, I teased myself, without my long and rambling sermons, everyone might forget about me!

The day after Christmas, the fatigue hit me with a full-body blow. I finally accepted that I needed some time off, maybe two weeks, and was almost ready to ask for it. I just needed to mount up my courage and make the call to the chair of our Staff Parish Relations Committee (personnel team).

Over the years, a few Bible verses had become familiar comrades in the battle for rest. I returned to them for insight.

"By the seventh day God had finished the work he had been doing; so, on the seventh day, he rested from all his work" (Genesis 2:2).

After a week of creative work, the most amazing work of all time, God rested. Even God takes a break.

Additionally, Adam and Eve rested with God. God created Adam and Eve on the final and sixth day of creation, and they all rested on the seventh day. That means the first task God gave to the first human beings was to rest. Rest is a priority. God hardwires the need for rest into our DNA. We work out of our rest.

The Bible instructs us, "Remember the Sabbath day by keeping it holy. Six days you shall labor and do all your work, but the seventh day is a sabbath to the Lord your God. On it, you shall not do any work" (Exodus 20:8-11).

This is number five on God's Ten Commandments. Work six days and rest one. God commands it.

More than a law, it's a gift. Sabbath provides a life-sustaining rhythm and model for living. Every week, we need a day to rest. Every day, we need some time to rest. Every year, we need some time away from work. We need Sabbath in our lives, and God gives it to us.

God provided for Sabbath rest for the fields farmed year after year. Even the fields need times of rest to replenish the nutrients and recapture the conditions necessary to produce another abundant harvest.

God wants all of creation to rest, every person, and everything. The commandment covers animals. "Six days do your work, but on the seventh day do not work, so that your ox and your donkey may rest" (Exodus 23:12). If God cares about donkey's resting, God certainly wants us to rest.

The Scripture also reminded me of the impact of Sabbath-keeping on my family's well-being and others connected to me.

One of my favorite verses says, "God gives rest to his loved ones" (Psalm 127:2, NLT). On many sleepless nights, I reminded God of his promise.

Now I sensed God offering me much more than a few hours. As I struggled to accept that I needed to rest and request some time off, more than any other, my heart returned to these words of Jesus.

> Are you tired? Worn out? Burned out on religion? Come to me. Get away with me, and you'll recover your life. I'll show you how to take a real rest. Walk with me and work with me—watch how I do it. Learn the unforced rhythms of grace. I won't lay anything heavy or ill-fitting on you. Keep company with me, and you'll learn to live freely and lightly
> —(Matthew 11:28-30, TM).

Jesus' invitation spoke to the depths of my being. Jesus knew I needed the rest, and he knew how hard it was for me to ask. I felt his assurance that he would show me the way. He would use my cancer and my fatigue to teach me how to rest.

Stymied and unable to make the call, I went to see my long-time counselor, Jane Clark. She welcomed me with a smile and led me into her office. I took my usual seat on the sofa. She knew me well, but we hadn't talked in a while.

After updating her on my health, family life, and other demands, I told her about my busy work schedule. I confessed that I really felt tired. I was even thinking I might take some time off from my job. As I rambled on, she took her standard copious notes while often looking over the rims of her glasses at me with a disconcerting look.

I told her about my continued exercise and long runs. According to my doctors, exercise was the best remedy for fatigue. I enjoyed running on the trails in the forest near our house. I also had several routes through town. I tried to run at least three miles every other day or two. Occasionally, I ran longer distances, like my eight-mile run this past weekend.

With an incredulous look, Jane Clark smacked her pad of paper on her lap, lifted her hand, signaling for me to stop, slid her glasses down to the end of her nose as she leaned over towards me, looking me dead in the eyes, and pointing her pen at me.

"You ran eight miles?" she asked in stunned disbelief.

"Yes. I'm thinking about a half-marathon."

"You ran eight miles. You went to how many meetings? You didn't take a day off?"

Her voice started soft and stern, but quickly grew to that of an exasperated parent trying not to yell at her kid.

"Of course, you're tired. You have stage four lung cancer! You aren't taking care of yourself. You aren't resting."

She stood up, walked over to me, took my hand in hers, leaned down to where her face was just a few inches from mine, and looked me right in the eyes. Speaking directly to my soul, she whispered, "Young man, if you keep this up, you will be resting… in the hospital or the morgue."

She let the words hang in the air for a few long seconds, never taking her eyes off mine before she squeezed my hands, patted me on the shoulder, shook her head one last time, and returned to her chair.

She had gotten my attention.

After a few minutes of discussing some of my psychoses that could be standing in my way, Jane Clark got straight to the point.

"When will you be taking time off?"

"I don't know. Soon, I think."

Unappeased with my answer, I sensed a new tactic.

"Open up your phone…yes, now…and find three weeks you can take off in January. Tell me the dates."

She leaned back in her chair, crossed her legs, and waited as I did as instructed. After flipping through my calendar, I reported one week I could take.

"That's not good enough. One week is not enough. You need at least three. Four, ideally."

I looked again at my calendar, considering the meetings I could miss, the couple Sundays I could have someone else preach, the responsibilities I could delegate to others, and the relative lightness of my schedule for January, and identified three weeks.

"Who needs to approve your request?"

"Only the chair of our Staff Parish Relations Committee."

"Call her right now. I want you to call her before you leave my office. Get it set up right now."

"Now?"

"Yes, right now."

I dialed the Chair and waited as the phone rang. Truthfully, I had wanted to ask, but my fear had prevented me.

Surprisingly, the Chair picked up. I made my request to take off three whole weeks. More surprisingly, she approved. It sounded like an excellent idea to her. She'd let the rest of the team know, and anticipated their full support. I thanked her and ended the call. Simple as that.

I looked over at Jane Clark as she leaned back into her chair with a smile on her face and applauded me lovingly.

Not only did the committee support me, on my last Sunday before my three weeks of Sabbath started, they asked me to join them at the front of the sanctuary in worship so they could pray a special blessing over me.

On the way home that day, I told one of my church friends that I had a problem: "I'm not sure I know how to rest. What would I do with my time off?"

"You know," he said, sarcastically, "you talked about that in your sermon a few weeks ago, about Sabbath rest. That was a great sermon. Maybe you should go back and listen to it."

Ouch. I hate it when that happens.

I took my friend's advice. It was a great sermon. Truly inspiring. I had included a couple of things I had learned from a book called *The Sabbath* by a famous Jewish Rabbi named Abraham Joshua Heschel. I had read the book a few years earlier, and a couple of things had stuck with me ever since.

First, Rabbi Heschel said, "Call the Sabbath a delight to the soul and a delight to the body."[7]

I dreaded being away from work. I worried I wouldn't enjoy it. I wouldn't know what to do. I might get in trouble for not working. I would miss my work. If I planned to rest, I would need an attitude adjustment. My Sabbath rest *would* be a delight. I *would* enjoy it. This time of renewal, refreshment, and restoration would be a delight.

Secondly, the Rabbi said, "Sanctify the Sabbath by choice meals, by beautiful garments; delight your soul with pleasure..."[8]

As I broke that down, a vision for my time off emerged.

To sanctify the Sabbath and my time off meant "to set apart" that time for God. A Sabbath day is a holy day. My three weeks would be sacred and holy. That alone made it special and joyful. Like the Sabbath day, I needed to protect, honor, and allow nothing to take it away from me in full or in part. This would be a special time with God and God's gift to me. Also, this time mattered to God. God had set it apart to be with me. It was on God's calendar.

Sanctifying my sabbath with "choice meals" sounded good. During my time off, I could delight in delicious meals. I could take off the shelf the cookbook my mother gave me at my wedding, the three ring-binder stuffed with the recipes she had made while I was growing up. I could prepare some of my favorites for my family and friends. I could take them all on a trip to "Flavortown," as Guy Fieri likes to say. Man cannot live on frozen pizza and chicken nuggets alone. During my sabbath rest, we could feast on the likes of Swedish meatballs, snickerdoodle cookies, and maybe even a bowl of "Michael's Favorite Rice Pudding." We could go to our favorite restaurants, eat our favorite foods, and delight our taste buds.

Wearing my "beautiful garments" would prove to be more challenging. One look at my side of the closet showed I didn't have any beautiful garments. I saw my twenty-five-year-old, go-to blue sport coat. I'll never forget smelling something awful at a district pastors meeting and discovering it was my jacket and that our cat had peed on it.

Looking at the multiple pairs of jeans with holes in the knees, worn-out and out-of-style shirts and ties hanging around after years, and an old tuxedo my dad gave me that I would never fit into, I knew what I had to do. My wardrobe looked like me—worn out. I had seldom taken the time to take care of me. I would have to go where no man wants to go—the mall.

I would need to get a new sport coat, shirt, pants, and a few other things. It occurred to me that as much I appreciated seeing my wife dressed up and looking extra beautiful, she might enjoy seeing me wearing something nice occasionally. Who knows? We might even have to go on a date!

In terms of delighting my soul with pleasure, I had to stop and think. I needed to remember what brought me delight besides work and my family. I have always delighted in writing. I have always loved to read. In college, I was enthralled with Jack Kerouac's *On the Road*. I was ready to hitchhike and ride trains across the country. I have always delighted in listening to music. I used to play the guitar and sing, and even write songs every day. Now I couldn't remember the last time I had picked up my guitar.

My weekend getaways with Amy delighted me. Spending time with her, our kids, family, and friends, my devotional time with God, and writing about my experiences of God. These were just a few of my favorite things, and I could incorporate them all into my sabbath rest.

Finally, Rabbi Heschel gave a short list of activities to avoid on the Sabbath. These Sabbath-sabotaging activities are prohibited. Number one: do not work on the Sabbath. That includes talking or thinking about work—no work calls, texts, or emails. Number two: Don't do, think, or talk about anything that causes you anxiety. No paying bills and balancing your checkbook or reviewing your homeowner's insurance policy. Number three: Don't pick a fight, even if it's a matter of right and wrong. Don't argue. (That's work!) Don't be angry on the Sabbath. Last: Don't be sad. All of this will wreck your rest.

With all the insights I had gleaned from the Rabbi, I embarked upon my three-week sabbath. I followed his advice as closely as I could. After a couple of days, I could earnestly call my sabbath a delight.

The last week of my leave, I spent at the beach by myself. A parishioner had offered me his "little place" on the North Carolina Outer Banks. Now being the off-season, his condominium was empty, few people would be around, and I could enjoy some solitude.

I decided my time at the beach would be a spiritual retreat. I planned to rest and reflect on God's presence in my life, especially over the past eighteen months of cancer. I took my Bible, my guitar, a notebook, my laptop, and a couple of books to read. I did not bring any church work or plan to do any. I also imposed a no-TV rule and limited my cell phone use to checking in once a day with Amy. I packed my beautiful garments and a small cooler of food for a few simple yet choice meals and headed for the beach.

My friend's place turned out to be an enormous six-room condo with an ocean view, and it was just a two-minute walk to the beach. The mornings I devoted to meditation, prayer, reflection, Scripture reading, journaling, and singing songs of worship. I enjoyed sitting on the sofa with a delicious cup of coffee in hand, with the porch door opened, watching and listening to the ocean and feeling the breeze. I spent the afternoons writing, working on this book, and reading. Throughout the days and evenings, I spent time on the beach—walking, exploring, picking up shells, running for exercise, and sometimes just staying still and practicing being present before God.

My devotional time each morning opened with a prayer and meditation. "Speak Lord, your servant is listening" (1 Samuel 3:9). I sat in silence for as long as I could stand it, trying to listen. I waited, awake, and aware, ready to hear what God might say and feel his presence. To the best of my ability, I emptied my mind and waited for what the Spirit brought to my mind. When something seemed Spirit-inspired, I scribbled it down in my notebook.

Each day brought something new. One day centered around gratitude for God's faithful provision. I could rest because I knew God would provide all I needed. Memories of all the generous people flooded my mind and my heart.

Another day focused on strength. I drew strength from God's power. Watching the ocean waves mounting up, rolling majestically, and crashing down testified to God's power. I understood that taking time to rest wasn't a sign of weakness. It was the source of strength.

On another, mercy moved to the center of my mind. I thought of how merciful God had been to me, and of all the people who had shown me kindness. "The steadfast love of the Lord never ceases; his mercies never come to an end. They are new every morning. Great is your faithfulness" (Lamentation 3:22). To rest is to have mercy on one's self.

On the last and most precious day, as I prepared to meditate, I waited in silence, struggling to empty my mind, and focused on the sound of the ocean surf. I thought about a prescription I needed to fill, bills I needed to pay, and other worldly affairs. Finally, three words came to mind—technically, four: peel 'n eat shrimp!

After I promised myself shrimp soon, three more words emerged—do not worry. I could hear Jesus' gentle rebuke: "Therefore I tell you, do not worry about your life, what you will eat or drink; or about your body, what you will wear."

I opened my Bible and read the rest of the passage. "Is not life more than food, and the body more than clothes? Look at the birds of the air; they do not sow or reap or store away in barns, and yet your heavenly Father feeds them. Are you not much more valuable than they? Can any one of you by worrying add a single hour to your life?" (Matthew 6:26-27).

I breathed in deeply the word "don't," held it, and then slowly exhaled "worry." I repeated this several times, turning the words into a prayer.

Cancer had given me a lot to worry about over the past eighteen months, and I had no idea what the future would hold for me. I did know, as cliché as it may sound, the One who holds my future. God didn't want me to be anxious or worry. God wanted me to trust him to continue to provide everything I needed to face cancer and my life.

In that time, I was reminded of a profound truth prerequisite to any rest. I could only rest and would only rest when I truly believed the Lord would faithfully take care of me. With faith in God, I could relax my heart, mind, and maybe even my body. I could rest secure.

On my last night, I treated myself to a Low Country Boil. I got the shrimp I had promised myself, and a whole lot more. I lifted the lid of the steamy red pot, leaned in, and looked over to see the mouthwatering, succulent crab legs, steamed shrimp, links of delicious assuage sausage, corn on the pod, and new potatoes. Taste and see that the Lord is good, y'all!

After three weeks off from work, I felt rested and ready to get back to work. On my last day at the beach, I took some time to envision the exciting ministries ahead. While I did look forward to the work ahead, I hoped God would continue to teach me to rest.

Trust

Two days after returning from my beachside sabbath, I learned that the Staff Parish Relations Committee had decided the church needed a new senior pastor.

The news shocked me and left me speechless. I heard the words, but I couldn't feel anything. Like someone who had just suffered a severe bodily injury—like losing a limb, maybe—I was in total shock and felt nothing.

The committee's Chair told me the conversation about a possible change of leadership came up unexpectantly at the committee's meeting while I was away. Committee members had come to believe that my cancer had diminished my performance as a pastor. They felt that my preaching and leadership were not as good as they had been. All agreed the church needed a pastor functioning at 100 percent.

The committee assured me that its decision also came out of concern for me. They worried about my well-being. Trying to serve as a pastor of a large and demanding church, on top of dealing with cancer, would be too much for anyone.

At their meeting, the matter had been discussed at great length. A motion had been made, the committee had voted, and the decision had been finalized. The "higher-ups" had been notified, as protocol required, and they were supportive.

Just like that, my fate was sealed. In three months, I would no longer be their pastor.

I was shocked. I had received so much love from the congregation. The Staff Parish Relations Committee had been supportive and given me positive reviews. My worst fears had come true.

A few days later, I pleaded my case to the bishop, the leader of our conference of several hundred churches. She alone had the final decision. She had always been supportive of me, believing in me and promoting me, and she cared about my family.

She listened empathetically, admitting mistakes had been made. Nonetheless, she made it clear the decision would stand. I had two options—take another church, probably smaller, or go on medical leave, aka disability, for a couple of years or longer.

She recommended medical leave as the best option. It would allow me to choose where I wanted to live and do what I wanted to do. I could use the time to take care of myself and be with my family. Moreover, medical leave would be most likely better for our family financially, given the churches that might be available.

With our meeting concluded, she stood up, reached across the conference table, and took my hand in hers. Looking directly into my eyes, she smiled sincerely, nodded her head affirmingly, and offered these parting, and perhaps prophetic, words, "Go write your book."

A few days later, I still wasn't ready to let go of my job. I consulted with an attorney friend of mine experienced in employment law. I thought there might be some legal way to get my job back. Over Chinese food, my friend gave me some free council. It didn't sound like I had much of a case. Employment laws regarding discrimination don't apply to churches like they do to others. Plus, I had signed up and agreed to serve wherever I was sent. Technically, I wasn't being fired; I was being appointed to another church or medical leave.

As we wrapped up, I opened my fortune cookie and read it out loud. "You are about to spend some time on the bench." *Are you kidding me?*

Later, I showed the little slip of paper to Amy, and she read the message back to me. "'You are about to spend some time on the beach.' It says beach, not bench. You're about to spend some time on the beach!"

We both got a good, and greatly needed, laugh out of my mistake. I did need to get some glasses. But beach or bench, either way, it sounded like I might be headed to medical leave.

The committee's decision devastated my family. We loved our church. We had made lots of friends. Many had become like family. We loved being in Chapel Hill—the schools, the people, the amenities, and the city's vibe. We had all envisioned our future there. We loved and appreciated the home the church provided us, the parsonage. Now, it all seemed to have been taken away.

I worried myself sick wondering what this would do to Amy and the our children's faith. They were so hurt. They might never come back to church. Who could blame them? Most importantly, I feared this would harm their relationship with God.

To see me, their beloved father and husband, dismissed and hurt, pained them. Amy had never fought harder for me. She believed in me and in my ministry. She couldn't stand to see it taken away. It was wrong and had to be made right. My children worried about me. Caleb, just fourteen years old, was upset and concerned about what this would do to my self-confidence. One day, out of the blue, he put his hand on my shoulder and offered words of reassurance. "Dad, I hope you know you're a great pastor."

I had thought I would be my church's pastor for many years. I loved it. I had even thought I might want to be buried in the church's cemetery if they could squeeze me in. Now, I questioned whether I would even be a pastor again, if there would be room for me anywhere.

In the days and weeks to follow, my mind and heart and emotions spun wildly. How could they? Cancer is hard enough. How would my family ever recover? Could I? What would this mean for us financially? We were just starting to get on our feet.

What would become of my life? More importantly, who would I be if wasn't Pastor David? I had just lost so much.

As my life began to settle down, I began to look for God's purpose in all that had happened, and in the uncertain future ahead. I had claimed by faith, from the start of my cancer journey, that God would use my cancer to glorify him. I believed that God was using my cancer to cure me. Now I wondered what healing could come from losing my job and being thrust into the unknown. As I asked and listened, the word *trust* continued to come to mind. I could hear God calling me to trust him.

One morning, in my devotional time, the Lord led me to this passage of Scripture in which St. Paul recounted some of his painful ministry experiences and how God used them to increase his trust in God.

"Brothers and sisters, you need to know about the severe trials we experienced...All the hardships we passed through crushed us beyond our ability to endure, and we were so completely overwhelmed that we were about to give up entirely. It felt like we had a death sentence written upon our hearts, and we still feel it to this day. It has taught us to lose all faith in ourselves and to place all of our trust in the God who raises the dead" (2 Corinthians 1:8).

Paul's words pierced me. Yes, of course, God would use this challenging experience to teach me to lose all faith in myself and place all my trust in God. God would use losing my job to help me gain more trust in him. God would use this loss to increase my trust in him. *Ok, God, I'm listening.*

Not surprisingly, God led me to many more verses related to trusting God. What I did not expect was how many of the Bible's messages were about who and what *not* to trust. As the saying goes, "Be careful who you trust."

First and foremost, the Bible says, whatever you do, don't put your trust in yourself. "Those who trust in themselves are fools" (Proverbs 28:26a). Several similar verses together give us a fuller understanding of what this means. Don't put your trust in your wealth, possessions, strength, understanding, or the works of your own hands, and even your own knowledge.

"Do not trust upon the wisdom of your soul" (Proverbs 3:5, Aramaic Bible in Plain English).

The Bible also tells us not to put our trust in other human beings. "Do not put your trust in princes, in human beings, who cannot save" (Psalm 146:3). The Bible makes a special point to warn against trusting those in power, in positions of prestige and influence, and leaders. If they cannot save us, everyday people certainly cannot either.

After putting all of this into one composite, it didn't take long to see the root of the problem. I had trusted in myself. I had undoubtedly trusted in the works of my hands. I had also trusted in others, including the Church and its leaders. I had given myself and others the trust that belonged to God alone.

I trusted if I did a good job, as close to perfect as humanly possible, I would continue to have financial security and keep moving up in the ranks. Maybe even more importantly, I trusted that the members of my church and others would give me my much-needed affirmation. "Great sermon, Pastor David." Their compliments and positive feedback made me feel loved, valuable, energized, and secure.

I trusted the church to provide my identity. In doing my work of serving them, I knew who I was—Pastor David. That was my purpose and my reason for living. I had fallen into a trap I knew all too well. I had been the victim of the worst kind of identity theft. So caught up in being a pastor, I had forgotten that I am, first and foremost, a beloved child of an awesome and loving God, saved by grace through faith in Jesus Christ.

I could hear the Father proclaiming, over Jesus, "This is my Son, whom I love; with him I am well pleased" (Matthew 3:17). I knew God spoke the same words to me. I knew God loved me and was pleased with me with or without the job, on or off disability. God loved me just the same. I could trust God for my purpose, affirmation, the provision of all my needs, and my identity.

Having my job taken away and possibly taking a couple of years off from parish ministry might prove to be precisely what I needed to redirect my trust and place it all in God.

I thought of a former parishioner of mine. One of the most truthful and trustworthy people I had ever known, who in her own cancer experience, demonstrated remarkable trust in God.

I met Karen while serving as one of the pastors at her church. As the associate pastor, I was responsible for the annual confirmation class—religious training the church provided for middle schoolers. Karen and her husband, Alan, had served as confirmation mentors for many years. Karen had been a guidance counselor for thirty years at a nearby high school. The students trusted her to always tell them the truth and want the best for them. Karen and Alan were mature, faithful Christians, and I enjoyed working with them.

One day, Karen and Alan came to me and shared the terrible news that she had been diagnosed with breast cancer. It was advanced and had already spread to her lymph nodes. Doctors scheduled her to have a double mastectomy, which would be followed by chemotherapy and radiation. They shared their concerns and hopes, and we prayed together.

On the day of the surgery, I joined them and their daughter, Alison, at the hospital and waited with them in the prepping area. Doctors had prepped Karen with IVs and monitors. I can see her now, lying on her gurney, tucked under the white blanket, wearing a blue surgical cap and a bright smile on her face. I offered words of encouragement, shared a promise of Scripture, and offered a prayer.

The nurse came to take Karen to the operating room, and we followed her down the hall toward the double doors, shouting words of encouragement. As the doors opened, I yelled, "Everything will be fine, Karen. I will see you on the other side."

Everyone stopped, even the nurse pushing the gurney, and looked at me in disbelief. Karen lifted her head and looked at me with big eyes. Alan and Alison looked, too, with the I-can't-believe-you-said-that look. Then all at once, they burst into laughter.

Embarrassed, I hurried to clarify: "I'll see you on the other side *of the surgery*." Gradually, I joined in their laughter. Karen laid back on the gurney with a big smile on her face, and the nurse rolled the gurney on into the operating room.

I was very grateful for their trust in God. Without it, they might not have been laughing. Karen might have erupted into tears. Alan might have knocked me out. Alison would have chased me out of the hospital. My unfortunate double entendre may have gotten me in serious trouble.

After recovering from the surgery, Karen started on chemotherapy. The powerful drugs took their toll. All too soon, Karen's red hair had fallen out. Her face had thinned. She had lost lots of weight as she had grown increasingly noxious and fatigued. After a few months in which we thought she might be improving, doctors reported that the cancer had spread. Meanwhile, chemo became intolerable.

Alan asked me to come over to the house and visit. When I entered the room, Karen smiled brightly at me. It seemed out of place in a room cluttered with a hospital bed, an IV and a morphine pump, an oxygen hose attached to her nose, and other medical equipment. I found her smile and laughter comforting. She looked angelic. Alan sat beside her, holding her hand.

I sat, and Alan handed me a note Karen had written. I read her words out loud: "No more chemo. We have to trust God to fulfill his promises. If we say we believe, then we have to show that we do. God asks us to trust him, love him, and accept his Son Jesus Christ. Follow him, love one another, and do as much good as we can. I have decided to follow Jesus. No turning back, no turning back."

Awed by Karen's trust in God, and deeply moved, I reached out, took her hand and Alan's in mine, and promised to continue to support them in the days ahead. Then we prayed together.

As we feared she would, she grew weaker. While her pain

intensified, she rarely showed it, at least not to me. She remained impossibly beautiful. She used the time to give her husband, daughter, grandchildren, and many others priceless assurances of her love, and received much love from them all. Although all too soon, she died peacefully with her husband and daughter at her side.

As I prepared for her funeral, I heard from many of Karen's former students and confirmands. One note included this commendation: "Karen was a mentor that I knew I could trust and go to for anything. And she taught me to trust in God's unending love and care."

Even now, many years later, Karen's witness still inspired me and challenged me. I, too, had a decision to make. Mine, fortunately, wasn't whether to continue fighting cancer with chemo or not. My choice was whether to fight to keep working or accept medical leave. Fighting against medical leave, like Karen's continued chemo, wasn't going to get me anywhere. My being angry, speculating motives, blaming others, and feeling betrayed hurt more than it helped.

It had been several weeks since the Staff Parish Relations Committee had let me go. I had come to believe that taking medical leave would be the best option, but I hadn't committed. I had begun to feel like I could use the time off and that it would be good for me. But I still didn't want to surrender.

One morning, in my devotional time, I read Psalm 32: "I will instruct you and teach you in the way you should go; I will counsel you with my loving eye on you. Do not be like the horse or the mule, which have no understanding but must be controlled by bit and bridle or they will not come to you. Many are the woes of the wicked, but the Lord's unfailing love surrounds the one who trusts in him" (Psalm 32:8-10).

The words smacked me on the backside. I could hear the Lord speaking to me: *Don't be like this mule...come with me.* I could sense God calling me to take this time of rest.

God may or may not have initiated the decision to take my job away or to push me onto medical leave, but God had allowed it, which meant God must have some useful purpose for it and would redeem the whole saga. These words of Scripture assured me of God's plan to use medical leave to care for my family and me and to evoke our trust in him. God would continue to demonstrate his trustworthiness.

Not comfortable with the idea of being eternally regarded by God as a stubborn mule, and more importantly, ready to place my trust in the Lord, I decided to take medical leave.

Some significant opportunities for trusting God soon appeared. We had about four months to prepare for medical leave, and a lot to do.

Two months after learning I would lose my job. I went in for my quarterly follow-up with my oncologist. It had now been six months since I had completed whole-brain radiation. So far, the results had been disappointing. At the first post-radiation follow-up, three months after completion of the treatment, I still had thirty or more tumors in my brain. If this follow-up didn't show far fewer tumors, I would likely be switched to a different chemotherapy drug, a new one that might be more effective in treating brain tumors like mine.

After the usual scans and lab work, Amy and I met with the oncologist, who shared the results. The scans were not better. A few of the previously seen tumors had gotten larger and moved dangerously close to my skull. This raised concern that the cancer could spread from my skull to my spine if it hadn't already. From there, it could spread everywhere...fast.

The news disappointed me and frightened me. My brain had been radiated eighteen times, with no apparent benefit. I could only imagine the unwarranted damage the radiation had caused my otherwise healthy brain. Only time would tell. Doctors ordered an MRI of my spine to be done at the earliest opportunity and scheduled another appointment. Until then, I would have to wait and continue to trust the Great Physician.

Fortunately, there was a lot to keep my mind occupied. For three months, we searched for a house and had no success. As much as we wanted to stay in Chapel Hill, we couldn't make it work. We expanded our search and finally found a house in Raleigh, and made an acceptable offer. At the last minute, the sellers decided not to sell the house.

I felt like giving up. We had found houses that were right but in the wrong place. Houses that were perfect, but sold before we got to them. Houses we loved, but couldn't afford. A rental that looked like a brothel, and worse. And now this!

As I had my meltdown, I remembered a Bible verse from my morning devotion: "Be silent and stop your striving and you will see that I am God" (Psalm 46:10a, TPT).

I took a moment and gathered myself and recommitted the search to the Lord. *No more striving. Show me what you've got, God.*

A minute later, Caleb came to me. A house had popped up on his cell phone. Unbeknownst to us, our fourteen-year-old had created a real estate search online. This house met all our specifications, which he had set up in his savvy query. Amy and I agreed, and we made an offer minutes later without seeing it in person. The offer was accepted.

The next day, we walked through the home and couldn't believe our eyes. It had everything we wanted. God, trustworthy and true, appeared to have dropped the house from heaven for us. We just had to trust God.

I prayed for grace at the bank when we applied for our mortgage. I doubted anyone would be excited to make a thirty-year loan to a middle-aged guy with stage four lung cancer. The Lord gave us a kind and helpful banker whose name happened to be Gracie. *Ok, God, now you're just showing off!* I asked for grace, and God gave us Gracie. With her help, we were approved for the loan and closed the deal right on schedule.

As we finalized preparations for our move, I planned to spend my last day in my office packing up and sorting through the thousand books—mostly unread—that stuffed my shelves. The reality of having no office to move my books to and no place in our home for them forced me to embark upon the long-overdue task of discarding half of my books, or more. I abhorred the idea of moving all these books again, especially the ones I knew I would never read.

The "Open Eye" four-shot espresso drink I picked up on the way to the church helped get me going along with the truckload of boxes Chuck and Alice had scored for me at the ABC store. My friend Adam's promise to swing by later with his big truck and help me haul my packed boxes wherever I wanted them to go also encouraged me.

As I sorted and packed my books and belongings into boxes marked "Keep" and "Discard," I couldn't believe how many I needed to discard. Or how many of those awful, and horribly heavy three-ring binders I had. I thought of how much energy I had expended hauling them through the years, their lack of worth to me, and the space they consumed. As I pondered, God gave me a vision.

Just as I wanted to discard these things, God wanted me to let go of some other things: the hurt and anger I felt over losing my job because of cancer; my regrets for what I could have done and what could have been; sorrow for those I would miss; my fears of what the future held for my family and me. Would my family be okay? Would I be a pastor again? Would I ever have a church office again? God wanted me to trust him with all this and more.

That afternoon, Adam and I discarded more than twenty-five bulging boxes. Throwing them into the dumpster was symbolic, cathartic, and even sacramental. I was letting go of my anger, fears, and other binders. I was giving up my trust in myself and everyone else, except God, who had again and again proved himself trustworthy and true.

As we headed back to my almost empty office, the wisdom writer's words filled my heart and mind, "Trust in the Lord with all your heart and lean not on your own understanding; in all your ways submit to him, and he will make your paths straight" (Proverbs 3:5-6, NIV).

Joy

On my first day of medical leave, I decided to go to my favorite coffee shop. I ordered a cappuccino and watched the barista pour the steamed milk into the espresso, magically making the frothy top look like a swan or a dragon, depending on your perspective.

I found a small table outside, between the shop's front window and the sidewalk. As I waited for my computer to boot up, I leaned back and looked at the bright and beautiful Carolina blue sky. The morning sun and a cool summer breeze felt good.

The morning went by quickly as I read, reflected, and typed away. After a few hours, I had the barista refill my cup. As he did, he asked me how I was doing. We chatted for a minute as I again marveled at his handiwork.

Back at my little table, I looked forward to my plans for the rest of the day. In that moment, I felt inspired to ask myself, *How am I doing?*

I didn't feel angry, sad, or depressed. For the first time in a long time, I didn't feel stressed. I felt peace. I felt grateful. I felt like medical leave might just be a gift in disguise. I felt excited.

I leaned back with my hands behind my head and a smile on my face. Dare I say it? I felt happy. I felt pure joy.

My happiness surprised me. This was my first day of being on medical leave. I had just been cut lose from my church.

I had cancer...in my brain. I probably should have been at home still, in bed, punching my pillow and crying my eyes out. Or maybe at the gym, taking out my anger on a punching bag. Not here sipping a superb cappuccino and smiling from ear to ear.

For most of my life, I would have considered myself a joyful person. I had a happy childhood filled with laughter and love. I was funny and could easily make people laugh. I enjoyed school. I tended to be the class clown, which my teachers probably didn't enjoy. My friends and I had a blast and tons of fun too many times to recall. My parents, my brothers, and I had plenty of family fun.

As an adult, I continued to be happy and experience joy. I had a beautiful, faithful wife. We had raised healthy, talented kids. I had friends, family, and meaningful work. I still found the funny things in life and made people laugh. In tense or boring work meetings, I could always loosen up the room.

Despite a lifetime of joy, over the past few years before my cancer diagnosis, I hadn't been feeling as joyful. Maybe the financial stress, the pressure to perform at work, the painful professional disappointments, or pressure in our marriage had been to blame. Or possibly all of it combined had put a damper on my happiness. Whatever was to blame, joy had become harder to find.

Sometimes I had felt apathetic; I just didn't care anymore. Other times, I had become hyper-critical and judgmental; nothing was good enough. All too often, my anger and resentment had snuffed out any possible joy. On too many mornings, I had put on my fake face and went to work.

I hadn't been able to hide the truth from my family. I can hear Amy, my fun-loving, life-is-good spouse, exasperated, asking me, "Do you like anything?"

"You second-guess every decision."

"Nothing is ever good enough for you."

"You take the fun out of everything."

My kids would even get in on the action: "Yeah, Dad, you're such a party pooper."

My cancer diagnosis was the proverbial straw that broke the camel's back. I wasn't sure how I would laugh or feel joy again. The diagnosis affected me like being fired from my job had. I don't recall ever shedding a tear over having cancer. It hurt too bad for me to cry. I couldn't feel anything for a while.

No one would have questioned me for being miserable. Most people would have expected me to be unhappy. Everyone knows that cancer is discouraging and depressing. If anything can pop your joy balloon, cancer can. Surely cancer would "wipe that smile right off your face."

Regardless of my assumptions and those of others, in a way, only God could, God had used cancer to help me rediscover joy, find new joy, and become more joyful than ever. I could see it as I looked back over the last eighteen months, since my diagnosis. And I knew in my soul; more joy was yet to come. To borrow a phrase from C.S. Lewis, I would continue to be "surprised by joy."

Fortunately, the Christian community specializes in joy. I went to church, and we still sang joyful songs like "Joyful, joyful, we adore Thee," "I've got that joy, joy, joy, joy down in my heart," and "He has made me glad."

We still preached and prayed about joy. I spent time with other Christians filled with joy. As surprising as many would find it, including myself, I felt some new joy.

The Bible has a lot to say about joy. During the early days and weeks after my cancer diagnosis, several passages of Scripture taught me about joy and helped me experience it in a fuller way.

To begin with, joy is found in the Lord. The Bible speaks of the "joy of the Lord" (Nehemiah 8:10c). Joy belongs to God. Jesus said if we are connected to him like a branch is to a vine, his joy will be in us and our joy will be complete (John 15:11). Joy is fruit produced in us by the Holy Spirit that Jesus gives those who believe (Galatians 5:22-23).

Joy is not human-made. God doesn't tell us to go and get happy, or to "turn that frown upside down." It's not up to us. God can fill us with joy in any circumstance, even during cancer.

Scripture shows us that joy is different from happiness. Joy is extreme happiness, sheer gladness, great pleasure or delight, and exhilaration. Joy defies definition. It's something inside that makes you want to "put your hands in the air and wave them like you just don't care!" It enables us to smile through the pain and dance in the rain. It gives us the deep satisfaction of having done what God desired of us.

Joy is how we feel and respond when God delivers us from trouble, provides for us in our time of need, shows us the way when we're perplexed, reveals himself through his works in our lives, and promises us a future with hope. It's the confidence of being assured of God's love and acceptance. Joy is that sacred something evoked when we give thanks for all God has done, when we truly worship, pray, and feast on his Word.

The Bible says, "The joy of the Lord is your strength" (Nehemiah 8:10c). In other words, it's more than a feeling. Joy is a power at work in us. According to one of my favorite Christian authors, Richard Foster, "Joy is the motor that keeps everything else going."[9] We all need joy to help us keep on trucking. No one needs the horsepower more than those living with cancer.

Believe it or not, joy can be experienced during cancer. The Bible often talks about joy in the context of pain and suffering.

"Consider it pure joy, my brothers and sisters, whenever you face trials of many kinds because you know that the testing of your faith produces perseverance" (James 1:2).

Because times of suffering and pain are often when our faith and our relationship with God grows the most, we can "consider it pure joy."

Psalm 30 testifies to the joy felt knowing the Lord will deliver you, and the joy experienced after the Lord has delivered you. While the Psalmist is sick and at death's door, he proclaims, "Weeping may last for the night, but rejoicing comes in the morning" (Psalm 30:5b). After the Lord has delivered him, he declares, "You (God) turned my wailing into dancing; you removed my sackcloth and clothed me with joy" (Psalm 30:11).

Truthfully, some of the most joyful people I know have suffered the most. Many were remarkably joyful in their suffering.

After my diagnosis, I thought of Janet, a former parishioner of mine. When I was her pastor, Janet was a sprightly seventy-five-year-old who looked and acted much younger. She was one of the most delightful little ol' ladies I had ever met, with her white hair, sparkling blue eyes, constant smile, and joyful demeanor. No one would have imagined her health challenges and journey.

Janet also had lung cancer that had spread and shown up in other places in her body. The last ten years of her life had been dominated by chemotherapy, radiation, biopsies, surgeries, hospital stays, reoccurring scans, doctors' reports, and all the rest. As if that weren't enough, she had also endured seven knee replacement surgeries to the same leg and needed another surgery. Tethered to a walker, her mobility had been severely compromised. She still found ways to stay connected and support the church, and I visited her often.

Despite all her struggles, I had never met a more consistently happy person. Janet was always thankful, optimistic, energetic, fun, and joyful. Every time we talked and I asked how she was doing, whether at the hospital, the church, or her home, she always had the same response, "Happy, happy." She even signed her emails and texts and letters, "Love, Janet Happy Happy."

When she could, she shuffled her way out of her single-level, all-flat senior living condo to her small car parked a few feet from her front door. On one such day, she met Amy and me for lunch. We greeted her at her car. "Hi, Janet, how are you?" True to form, Janet replied, "Happy, happy." As we took our seats, Janet brightened up the restaurant and our day.

Sadly, the location of our worship service, the distance from the parking lot, and the number of stairs made it almost impossible for Janet to come to worship most Sundays. I remember visiting her at the hospital on one Sabbath. She was lying on the gurney, in her gown. Even with the wires and tubes running every which way, and the monitors buzzing and blinking, she had a big smile on her face. She turned off the Joel Osteen sermon and welcomed me warmly. I asked how she was, knowing her answer.

"Happy, happy."

In one of our times together, Janet told me how she came to be so "happy, happy" even with cancer and all her other life and health challenges. She had been in the hospital for something else seemingly unrelated when doctors found the cancer. They came into her room after the surgery, reported that it went fine, but unfortunately, she had lung cancer.

Once the doctors left the room, she got out her Bible. Not knowing where to begin, she opened it on her lap, letting the pages fall wherever they would. After they had, Janet looked down and read these words:

> Rejoice in the Lord always. I will say it again: Rejoice!
> Let your gentleness be evident to all. The Lord is
> near. Do not be anxious about anything, but in every
> situation, by prayer and petition, with thanksgiving,
> present your requests to God. And the peace of God,
> which transcends all understanding, will guard your
> hearts and your minds in Christ Jesus
> —(Philippians 4:4-7).

At that moment, Janet experienced the presence of God and the peace that passes all understanding. She decided then not to be anxious, not to worry, but instead to rejoice and give thanks just like the Bible said. Trusting Jesus fully, she could be "Happy, happy."

One day, Janet texted me that she was not feeling well. She had lost her voice a few weeks earlier and still hadn't gotten it back. Diagnostic scans ordered by the doctors had raised some cancer concerns. She asked me to come over so she could share with me her funeral plans, something she had wanted to do for a while. She greeted me at the door of her apartment with her customary smile and mouthed the words, *Happy, happy.* We sat, and she handed me a couple of pieces of paper covered with lists of Scripture readings, song titles, and the customary components. The inclusion of the hymn "Joyful, Joyful, We Adore You" did not surprise me. It represented the theme of her life and seemed to be another way of saying "Happy, happy," which she had written in the margin.

Janet's testimony continued to inspire me and challenge me. I found her ability to rejoice with cancer and all her other challenges to be more miraculous than being cured of cancer. Every day, I wanted to be able to rejoice, no matter what. I wanted to be able to shout out, "Happy, happy."

Looking back on my cancer journey, I could see many ways I had experienced greater joy since being diagnosed. I found greater joy in being a dad. I had a blast moving Marcie into college and spending time with her on campus. She came home to celebrate her twentieth birthday a few months later. Two of her new college friends joined our family for dinner. Seeing Marcie so grown up, enjoying her friends, hearing her tell us all about school, and her new friendships brought me joy.

I loved seeing Hannah perform with her acapella group, cabaret choir, chorus, and musical theater productions. Even in a supporting role, she stole the show. I marveled at how our shy and reserved daughter turned into a superstar whenever she took center stage. Most of all, I loved watching her face light up when she performed. Seeing her camaraderie with her thespian friends only added to my joy.

Caleb landed a leading role as Link in *Hairspray*. The role of teenage heartthrob seemed custom-made for him, and I watched in awe as he sang, danced, and acted, and delivered a show-stopping onstage kiss to the leading lady before a packed house. He brought the house down, and he sent my joy through the roof.

My spirit soared when Marcie and Caleb led worship at our church. He would play guitar and sing. She would sing, too, and harmonize with him. The rest of the band encouraged them and brought out their best. Pure joy!

We celebrated Hannah's graduation from high school with a big bash. My Aunt Sharon and Uncle George flew in to join us for a fun-filled weekend. Caleb graduated from middle school, which wrapped up with a surprising amount of pomp and circumstance. Despite the rock-hard bleachers and an extremely long graduation service, I enjoyed that as well.

The Scripture reminds us, "Children are a gift from the Lord; they are a reward from him. Children born to a young man are like arrows in a warrior's hands. How joyful is the man whose quiver is full of them" (Psalm 127:3-5, NLT).

To that, I could truly say, *Amen!*

With cancer's help, I rediscovered joy in my marriage. When cancer showed up in my life, I wasn't enjoying my marriage. I wasn't happy. Cancer quickly put my complaints in check. Many people reached out, but Amy was the one standing beside me and with me every step of the way. To say I had a renewed appreciation for her would be a gross understatement. It was more like I had been reborn. I could see her beauty, strength, faithfulness, loyalty, courage, all the wonder of her, and more than anything, her love for me. As I let go of my anger, resentment, and all my negative feelings, I felt joyful and was overwhelmed by love for Amy.

Dear friends gifted us with a weekend getaway to Ashville, NC, amidst the Blue Ridge mountains. We made reservations at the charming bed and breakfast where we had stayed a few years earlier and thoroughly enjoyed ourselves and the hospitality. At check-in, the owners told us we had been bumped up to the wedding suite. Someone had canceled their reservation. Whether due to a change of vacation plans or cold feet, their loss became our gain. The suite suited us perfectly. We felt like newlyweds. Cancer had given us a new lease on life and our marriage. We could also benefit from the luxurious pampering and delicious breakfasts.

It was late fall, and we enjoyed driving and taking in the scenery, the changing colors of the foliage. One evening, we toured the Biltmore Estate, which had only recently been decorated for Christmas, making it even more special. We strolled through the historic mansion on a walking tour, hand in hand, taking in the splendor and glory of it—the humongous house made for an inescapably long tour. I don't think we had held hands that long since we first met.

We later capped off our time at Biltmore with a tour of its winery and a deliciously enjoyable wine tasting. Afterward, we walked out into the dark, into a spectacle of white lights strung from building to building, tree to tree, in all kinds of curious designs, creating a magical winter wonderland. Walking through a tunnel covered with an extended canopy of lights, I felt overwhelmed by the moment. Amy had never looked more beautiful. I had never felt more in love. We stopped and kissed, and I took pictures of the two of us that I will forever treasure, especially the one with Amy kissing me on the cheek. Pure joy!

In the days following medical leave, as my holy hunch had led me to believe, my joy continued to increase. Every day brought a little more happiness into my life.

The simple tasks of life brought me newfound joy. One morning, a few days into medical leave, I spent writing in my office at home. After lunch, I set out to run errands as planned: the ABC store for some more boxes, the thrift shop to drop off some stuff, the landfill to dispose of whatever the thrift shop wouldn't take, the home superstore for moving supplies, and lastly, the restaurant to order food for Hannah's graduation party.

With so many places to go, I expected it would take most of the afternoon. Hopefully, I could finish and be home before five o'clock traffic. The old me would have resented having to run all these errands. That day, as I cranked up my red minivan, pulled out of my driveway, looked up at the Carolina blue sky, and hit the gas, it felt like an adventure.

Racing across town, from one stop to the next, I remembered taking my dad's bright blue '72 Ford pickup truck out for a drive on the ten acres of pasture behind our house. The field sprawled out the size of two football fields. The freshly cut grass, the Carolina blue skies, the truck in the driveway with gas in the tank, the keys on the kitchen counter, and expecting no one home for a few more hours proved too tempting for a fifteen-year-old burning up to drive.

For an hour, I drove laps around the field and crisscrossed it. I practiced changing gears, mastering the timing between the clutch and the stick shift. I accelerated as fast as I could, shifting through the gears like a pro, listening to the engine roar. I slowed as I skidded through the corners. Leaned into the turns, rounded the corners as fast as I could, downshifting mid-turn, and then blasting off into the straightaway. I gripped the steering wheel with one hand, the shifter with the other, and shouted like one of the *Dukes of Hazzard*.

It was glorious until I saw my dad leaning against the fence, watching and waving for me to stop. His face was not nearly as joyous as mine. He had gotten home early, or I had lost sense of time. I don't remember what he said, but he wasn't happy. I, on the other hand, couldn't get the smile off my face. It had been an unbelievable joy ride.

Now, life seemed like a joy ride: writing for hours every morning, sipping cappuccinos at the café, and reading for pleasure. I enjoyed driving Amy to work and picking her up so she wouldn't have to deal with parking at the hospital. Purging and packing up our house and preparing for the move. Spending time with my kids and being part of their activities. Working out at the gym, swimming, going on vacation, and grocery shopping. It all brought me joy. I even found joy going to the cancer clinic— seeing my care team and hoping for a good report.

I discovered the joy of cooking. I took time to shop, and time to prepare meals. For breakfast, I often enjoyed yogurt parfaits—bananas and strawberries mixed with thick Greek yogurt and crunchy granola. Every few days, I'd splurge and make a three-egg omelet filled with cheese.

I enjoyed making myself lunch. I'll never forget one amazing strawberry walnut spinach salad. I chopped up the fresh green spinach, diced a little red onion and green pepper, dropped in a few bright red cherry tomatoes, sliced some juicy strawberries, chopped the walnuts, and mixed it all up. I topped it off with mozzarella cheese, and lastly, the strawberry vinaigrette dressing. *Bon Appetit!* The salad looked like a masterpiece work of art, a reminder of the beauty and goodness of God's creation. And it tasted delicious.

I dusted off the recipe book my mom gave me, filled with the foods I grew up on, and cooked some of my favorites—her homemade meatballs and meatloaf, chicken enchiladas, chicken crescents, and of course, snickerdoodle cookies.

I enjoyed cooking with chef Caleb, my son, who instituted Meatball Monday, Taco Tuesday, Weft-over Wednesday, and Smash-burger Saturday. Watching Caleb smashing the beef over the grill as it sizzled to perfection, mixing up his secret sauce, prepping veggies like a pro, and then crafting it all together into a burger that would rival any restaurant in town brought joy to my heart and taste buds. We made homemade pizzas, fettuccine alfredo and parmesan chicken, and so many other delicious foods.

One night, I was watching a television show featuring a home organizing guru famous for teaching people across the country and beyond how to "tidy up" their lives.[10] She directed her mentee, a young, overwhelmed mom, to make a pile of all her clothing in the center of the room. Seeing this Mt. Everest of clothing, the mentee couldn't deny she needed to get rid of a lot of it to tidy up. The guru then had her go through each piece, expressing gratitude to each for its service and asking herself if it "sparked joy" in her. In other words, did it give her a good feeling or make her smile. If it did not, it was folded and set aside in a pile to be given away.

The guru spent a lot of time teaching her student how to fold the clothing she chose to keep. I marveled at how she folded t-shirts into little four-inch by four-inch squares that were able to stand up on edge. Afterward, she packed them in the drawer, standing them upright instead of laying them flat so every shirt could easily be identified.

I followed her steps and organized my t-shirt drawer. *Wow! My mom would have passed out if I had done this as a kid.* So impressed with myself, I decided to remake Amy's t-shirt drawer. As I folded each of her two hundred t-shirts (perhaps a slight exaggeration), I didn't do any purging. I did thank God for her shirts and for Amy, who certainly sparked joy in me. Finished folding, I reloaded her shirt drawer. My handiwork said *I love you* more than two dozen roses would have, and I found great joy in doing it.

The exercise made me think about my life as a whole and some of the tidying up needed. I had so much joy-sparking stuff in my life, but it had been buried by my anger, unforgiveness, impatience, fears, anxieties, and workaholism. The transition to medical leave, the whole experience of cancer, my ministry, and my life had become one enormous heaping pile before me. I now had the opportunity to go through it all, piece by piece, and consider what did and did not spark joy.

As we made final preparations to move to Raleigh, North Carolina, the time came for my next quarterly checkup appointment with my oncologist. At this one, we would find out if cancer had gotten into my spine. The MRI and CT scan of my lung would also show us the state of the cancer in my brain and lungs.

I sat in the clinic and waited for the oncologist. He came in a few minutes later and pulled up the images on the computer for us to view. There had been some improvement in the brain, which was good news, but numerous tumors remained.

From that point, we talked mostly about the new chemotherapy I would begin immediately. Studies showed it to be more effective in the brain than what I had been taking. He listened to my lungs and checked me over, as usual. Everything looked good.

He stood, bid us well, and headed towards the door.

"Wait a second, Doc," I said. "What about the scan of my spine? Any cancer?"

"Oh, sorry about that. All of that looks perfectly normal. No cancer."

For the life of me, I didn't know why he hadn't started with that news and how he could forget.

With one foot out the door, he turned toward me and said, "I didn't think we needed that MRI, but radiology ordered it just to be safe."

I didn't know what else to say other than, "Happy, happy!"

Friendship

People say you never know how many friends you have until something bad happens to you. That was certainly true of my cancer diagnosis. Friends reached out from every direction. They flew in, drove in, emailed, sent cards, texted, and called. I heard from friends from middle school, high school, college, and graduate school. I heard from colleagues, mentors, pastors, and other important people. Parishioners from every church I had served or belonged to reached out.

When you have cancer, you also learn to appreciate your friends. You see how great they are and how much they mean to you. I could see that God had blessed me with many incredible friends.

My friend Thurman took a day off from his work as a busy pastor to go with me to my first MRI. He picked me up, drove me to the hospital, sat with me in the waiting room, prayed with me before the exam, took me to lunch afterward, and then drove me home. I probably would never have asked him to come, but I appreciated his being there with me. MRI's are unnerving, especially the first time, and especially when they're looking for cancer.

We met in pastors' school—boot camp for new pastors—almost twenty years earlier. In the years to follow, Thurman became one of my best friends. Honestly, I had never known a better friend. Like me, his ministry and life kept him ridiculously busy. Nonetheless, he always took the time to be a great friend. When our daughter, Hannah, was born, Thurman showed up to see us and meet her before our own families arrived. In difficult seasons of ministry, he supported Amy and me. He sent cards. He checked in. He prayed for us. When the cancer diagnosis came, he was there.

During that MRI, I prayed that God would help me be a better friend, more like Thurman. "Lord, use this MRI to rearrange my brain cells to make me a better Christian, a better parent, and a better friend." While I knew that transformation would need to happen in my heart, not just my brain, I felt an assurance God would use this cancer to make me a better friend and more appreciative of my friendships.

Days after my cancer diagnosis, Chris, whom I mentioned in the "Strength" chapter, and his wife, Lynn, dropped everything and drove several hours to spend the weekend with us. Their visit and our time together, especially our run through the woods, had given me a second wind.

Amy and I met Lynn and Chris about fifteen years earlier. They had recently moved to town and visited the church where I happened to be serving. Lynn and Amy met, quickly became friends, and thought our families should have lunch together after a Sunday worship service. Soon after, at a large table in a busy restaurant, Chris and I met. We hit it off and instantly became friends.

As our families continued to spend time together, Chris and I became confidants. After he finished his fellowship, he took a job in Ohio, and his family moved to Cleveland. Our families stayed in touch and visited one another a couple of times a year or more. His family visited us at Easter. We drove up from North Carolina to see them at Thanksgiving or Christmas.

Not long after their move, Chris and I endured professional challenges that for both of us resulted in an unexpected and challenging job change and family move. Through these hard times, he and I spent many hours on the phone talking and helping each other. I valued Chris's wise and caring words of encouragement and challenge. Through it all, we grew to be more like brothers than friends.

Among Chris's most admirable qualities is his generosity. One day, he literally gave me "the shirt off his own back," a beautiful brown suede jacket. He claimed he didn't need it and thought I might be able to use it. As I recall, my leather jacket at the time looked ragged. When Chris bought himself a new car after getting his first big-time job after finishing his fellowship, he gave me his old car, a vehicle much nicer than my car, which Chris knew needed repairs.

On so many occasions, when Amy and I visited them, we rode into town on fumes. For the first several years that we knew Chris and Lynn, Amy, and I struggled financially. We could barely afford to travel up, but we wanted to see them. Chris knew that and took care of every expense in a way that put me at ease. When the server at the restaurant brought the check, Chris wouldn't let me have it. Usually, I never saw it come to the table.

Chris filled our weekend visits with special activities— taking everyone to a trampoline park, ice skating, to the movies and out for pizza, or some other fun activity. I remember one of our visits to Cleveland that included, among other things, a visit to the Rock 'n Roll Hall of Fame, the museum, the zoo, and attending a Cleveland Indians' baseball game.

I could and should write a tribute to each of my many excellent friends. Cancer brought into sharp focus how much each meant to me. Cancer can make you feel alone. To be alone and facing such enormous uncertainties and challenges would be awful. I thanked God for Chris and others who called me to check on me. I praised God that I had friends who would listen to me and reassure me. As the song goes, "We all need somebody to lean on."

I used to think the opposite of a friend is an enemy. But the opposite of a friend is being alone. The opposite of being a friend is letting someone else be alone.

I've heard before that solitary confinement is the cruelest punishment. Some regard it as abuse or even torture. Being alone, especially in our struggles and pain, isn't healthy, and it's not God's intention. As I earlier referenced, after God capped off the glorious work of creation with the making of Adam, he pointed out creation's one flaw: "It is not good for the man to be alone" (Genesis 2:18). And so God created Eve to be Adam's partner...and friend.

Thinking about the significance of friends reminded me of a couple of Bible verses I discovered while teaching a class on Christian fellowship at one of the churches I served.

> *Two are better than one because they have a good return for their labor: If either of them falls, one can help the other up. But pity anyone who falls and has no one to help them up.*
> —(Ecclesiastes 4:9-10).

Never had I so appreciated having friends to pick me up and keep me secure.

Cancer also made me take stock of my childhood friends, some of whom I hadn't talked with in years. One by one, they contacted me just moments after hearing my bad news. As they did, encouraging memories abounded of elementary school, middle school, and high school.

Allen was my best friend growing up. We met in the sixth grade and had lots in common, including being newcomers to the same small town. We quickly became inseparable. In middle school, we found escape at his house after school, drinking Sun Drops, lip-syncing, and playing air guitars along to the likes of Hall and Oats and Air Supply. In high school, we had so much fun together, serving as the Statler and Waldorf of our school. We were just like those two Muppets in the balcony, cracking jokes and making fun of everything and everyone.

We started drifting apart as friends when girls and girlfriends became our focus. We were both on a mission to find "that lovin' feelin.'" Allen and I graduated and went to separate colleges. A few years later, each of us had found the love of our lives, got married, and started families. We worked hard and achieved success in our careers. Moves separated us geographically. Sadly, over the next thirty years, we spoke only a couple of times.

When Allen heard I had cancer, he reached out to me. As we caught up, we discovered both of us had been through some severe challenges since we'd last connected. To my surprise, he'd been through some potentially life-threatening stuff. We had needed each other but hadn't known. We both could have used a friend on many occasions. We recommitted to our friendship and to staying in touch.

Reconnecting with Allen struck a nerve. I hadn't been a good friend to Allen, let alone a best friend. It pained me to consider how many other friends I had lost touch with and what they might be going through. My call with Allen sounded the alarm.

Having so many friends reach out to me revealed that I needed to be a better friend. God had blessed me with several best friends over the course of my life, but had I been a best friend? Had I been as good of a friend as I should have been?

Maybe I was being too hard on myself. Nonetheless, when I looked back honestly at myself, I saw a friend who received more than he gave, responded more than he initiated, forgot more than he remembered, and didn't always show up.

I could blame it on my job. At the end of the day, there wasn't much left to give my family, let alone my friends. Changing jobs every few years made it harder. Of course, many other people managed to be successful in their careers and maintain close friendships. That included many of my friends who kept our relationships alive.

Looking ahead, I saw the opportunity to become a much better friend. Cancer could be a season of appreciating my friends, considering the meaning of friendship, being a better friend, and maybe even making some new friends. God could use my cancer to heal me of anything preventing me from being the best friend I could be.

The Bible contains many relevant verses demonstrating the importance of friendship. Friendship is a godly thing. God created us for it, and it empowers us.

One of my favorite stories of friendship is found in the Old Testament book of Ruth. The friendship of Ruth and Naomi is a beautiful example. Naomi, a widow, suffers the sudden loss of her two adult sons and is left with their fiancés. The three are alone in a culture where women depend on men for their livelihood. Naomi begs the two women to leave and go on with their lives, find men for themselves, and get married. One tearfully leaves Naomi to go home. The other, Ruth, refuses to leave Naomi, who begs her also to go. Ruth replied, "Don't urge me to leave you or to turn back from you. Where you go, I will go, and where you stay, I will stay. Your people will be my people and your God my God" (Ruth 1:16).

Theirs is a beautiful story of friendship that leads to redemption for all involved. Ruth finds and marries a kind and prosperous man, who takes her and Naomi in as part of his family.

The friendship between Jonathan and David resonates, especially as I reflect on my male friends. Jonathan was the son of Saul, the reigning King of Israel. During his reign, God called David to take Saul's place as king. Saul did not want to let go of his power and tried to dispose of David. Despite these more than hostile conditions, David and Jonathan became close friends. The two deeply connected, loved each other, wanted the best for each other, and put their lives on the line for each other. They made a covenant to support each other. "Jonathan became one in spirit with David, and he loved him as himself" (1 Samuel 18:1).

Upon Jonathan's death, David expressed his love for Jonathan. David lamented, "I grieve for you, Jonathan, my brother; you were very dear to me. Your love for me was wonderful, more wonderful than that of women" (2 Samuel 1:26). This isn't to say that husbands should love their wives any less. It does remind us of the importance of friends that love each other deeply.

Jesus' life and ministry contain many examples of friendship. Jesus himself had friends like Martha, Mary, and Lazarus.

Lazarus had become sick and died before Jesus had returned home and could save him. When Jesus saw Mary, Martha, and Lazarus' grieving friends, Jesus became emotional. The Bible records, "Jesus wept" (John 11:35). He cried because he cared, and he loved his friends. Fortunately for them both, Jesus had the power to raise Lazarus back to life.

If Jesus, the son of God, somehow both divine and fully human, needed friends, we can be sure we do as well.

Jesus thought of his disciples as friends. "I do not call you servants any longer, because the servant does not know what the master is doing; but I have called you friends" (John 15:15). Jesus was especially close to Peter, John, and James. Jesus taught his disciples how to love and be friends with each other.

God created each of us to be God's friend. Even if we haven't been a best friend to God, he remains our best friend. God sent Jesus to restore that friendship by giving up his own life for his friends. Jesus said, "No one has greater love than this, to lay down one's life for one's friends" (John 15:13).

When we are friends with God, we will have good friends and be a good friend. In fact, the closer we get to God, the closer we get to one another.

I knew all these Bible teachings and many more about the value of friendship. As I pondered them anew, I continued to sense God's desire to lead me to value friendship more and make me a better friend. As a cancer patient, held up in the arms of friends, the time had never been better.

The first couple of months of medical leave were a flurry of enjoyable activity. We moved into our new home and made it our own. We took a beautiful, much-needed family summer vacation. My cancer treatments continued to go well, and physically, I felt great. I devoted several hours each day to writing this book. I enjoyed the freedom to set my schedule, to exercise regularly, and to spend more time with my family. I enjoyed it all, but when life settled down to our new normal, I started feeling something I didn't usually feel—lonely.

I decided to call a few friends. I needed to talk, maybe even meet for lunch or coffee. One after another, each of my calls went straight to voicemail. I must have called six friends, and no one answered. I left messages saying I was thinking about them and wanted to catch up. No one responded. I got one text message, saying he'd call me ASAP. By the end of the day, I still hadn't heard from anyone.

Hearing from no one made me worry. With self-deprecating humor, I teased myself. *Man, oh man, I may be a worse friend than I thought! The world's worst!*

As I reflected, I started thinking about the vital role the church had played in almost all my friendships. I could remember the experiences and the many special friends I had made through my participation in the life of the church.

When my family moved from the sprawling suburbs of Charlotte, North Carolina, to the small country town of Locust an hour away, I knew no one. I was twelve years old. Unlike my old neighborhood where the houses were close together, and kids my age lived close by, our new home was far from all the others, and there were no kids in sight.

Soon after we moved in, my parents took us to a small, white A-frame country church not far from our house. The Presbyterian congregation greeted us warmly at the door. *Yes, we would be happy to stay after for the monthly fellowship lunch.* To this day, I can see my mom looking over her shoulder and giving my younger brothers and me "the look."

In the sanctuary, a few boys sat together in a pew near the front of the sanctuary. They saw me, and seconds later, one of the older boys, James, came over and invited me to sit with them. They were all a few years older and so cool. I followed their lead as they bowed to pray, stood up to sing, and tried to pay attention to the sermon. After the service, at lunch, they got to know me and invited me back for youth group. Just like that, I went from feeling like nobody to the king of the world. I had some cool friends.

Every church I have ever belonged to has welcomed me. Upon each new arrival, God seemed to have put in place at least a few friends chosen for me. Being a pastor gives you the fast pass, but all the churches I've served have had ministries and people ready and wanting to befriend all who came. It saddens me, and surely the heart of God, to know so many people don't feel accepted or wanted by the church.

As I pulled our minivan into the parking lot of the second church I was assigned to serve, for our introductory visit, I felt overwhelmed. With its high steeple towering over the surrounding neighborhood and the entire full-block edifice made of gothic stonework, it looked like a Roman cathedral. I had been assigned to serve this two-thousand-member congregation as the associate pastor, the second-in-command.

After our introductory visit with the Staff Parish Relations Committee, Amy and I pushed our baby stroller and transported our two young daughters through a busy hallway from the education wing, where the children had been occupied, and to the gymnasium-sized fellowship hall for church's Wednesday evening fellowship dinner. Seemingly hundreds of people moved through the crowded hallway, many others with children in tow, and poured into the fellowship hall, some peeling off into the food line. Others scattered off to find a table.

We followed the young woman our age, whom we met after the meeting, to a table full of young adults with families like ours. As we came through the crowd, the table seating prepared for our family came into view. Several young couples with their children stood around a long table to welcome us. They hugged us like they had known us their whole lives. For the next hour or more, we talked, laughed, and fellowshipped. In those moments, we met several life-long friends, including Ashley and Susan, who would come to my bronchoscopy fifteen years later.

As I served larger churches, I spent more and more time in "small groups." These gatherings of a dozen people, sometimes more and other times less, focused on growing in Christian faith together and providing an opportunity for members to make faithful friends.

I can recall arriving at the cute bungalow for the women's small group I was helping launch. Each week, the group of six ladies took turns hosting and providing a simple lunch. Most were new to our church. Each wanted to connect with others and grow in their faith.

At the front door, Lacy welcomed me with an enthusiastic, "Brother David!" She ushered me into her kitchen, where lunch awaited, and the rest of the group had already gathered.

As we sat together at Lacy's dining room table, we took turns sharing about our lives. We talked about our personal Bible reading since our last meeting. We focused on how we had sensed God speaking to us in the week before and how we should respond. The women spoke about marriage, children, and work. As Lacy was sharing, she started to cry, and the others comforted her. We finished our time with prayers for each other and a piece of Lacy's homemade cake.

In many times like these, I witnessed friendships being made. I also made many friends, some of whom I'm still close to and love, including sister Lacy.

In small groups like these, I learned the most about being a Christian friend. As I reflected on such groups, I thought of four key characteristics of friendships.

1. Friends want the same thing, the best for each other. They help each other attain their full God-given potential. The wholeness and happiness of the one depends upon the other fulfilling his or her deepest desires. Friends lay down their lives for each other (John 15:13).

2. Friends "speak the truth in love" (Ephesians 4:15). They share honestly and lovingly with each other about their lives. They each confess where they might be falling short. They also share how they see the other falling short.

3. Friends hold each other accountable and provide mutual support. They help each other name what needs to change and claim the power of Christ. They confess their sins to one another (James 5:16).

4. Friends "bear each other's burdens" (Galatians 6:2, ESV). They sacrifice and show up for each other, and above all else, love each other. They listen, help, and pray for each other.

Friendships such as these are a rare and priceless gift. Christian friendships are different from other relationships we have, and certainly, from the online social media experiences with people, we call friends. Having so many genuine Christian friends made my heart glad and inspired me to want to be a better friend.

As I looked back at the churches I had grown up in and served, I saw many friends. Inez, a former parishioner, a wise and wonderful older saint, had once told me, near the beginning of my ministry, "Some friends are for a season, some are for a reason, and a few are forever." Her sage wisdom had proven to be true. Wherever I lived, at every stage of my life, whatever I might have been doing, I always had great friends. *Thanks be to God!*

As I reminisced, I had an epiphany. Yes, I needed to be a better friend. I also wanted to appreciate my friends more. And I needed to be reminded of what Christian friendship is all about. I could see God using cancer to help me grow in each of those ways. But I also recognized that a big part of feeling alone came from my not belonging to a church family for the first time in my life.

Healing

Janice entered my office and took a seat. I hadn't expected her and had no idea what might be on her mind. I recognized her as one of the older members of my church, although I didn't know her well. She seemed quiet and reserved.

Janice expressed her heartfelt concern for my recent diagnosis with stage four lung cancer and asked how I was doing. After a brief update, she handed me a small bottle of ointment.

"I don't do mammograms," Janice said. "I don't believe in them. Whenever I feel a lump on my breast, I just put some of this ointment on it. I've never had any problems."

Janice laid on my desk what appeared to be a small newspaper. I picked it up and surveyed the headlines, pictures, and stories about how the ointment had healed people of all kinds of ailments, including cancer.

I thanked Janice for caring and sharing the ointment with me. Although I felt comfortable with the Duke Cancer Clinic and mainstream, traditional medicine, I promised to give the ointment a try. *Who knows?* I thought to myself. *I might rub some on my chest right after you leave. What have I got to lose?*

After my diagnosis, from the start, I received many precious prayers for healing, and messages wishing me well. I also received many treatment suggestions. If anyone knew of a potential cure, they told me about it.

One swore by a cancer-killing diet. "Cut out the sugar and starve the cancer to death!" Skeptical and a serious sugar lover, I had to pass. Some stressed the importance of positive thinking. I doubted that would be enough. Others sent me information about cutting edge medical breakthroughs and highly effective cancer treatments, which encouraged me greatly. The differing approaches shared one thing: the desire for me to be healed.

In the Bible, there are many stories of physical healing. We find some in the Old Testament and many more in the New Testament. As a long-time Christian and pastor, I had heard them many times. After being diagnosed with cancer, every account of healing took on new meaning.

Healing was central to Jesus' ministry and primary to his proclamation of the Good News of the Kingdom of God. He restored sight to the blind, cleansed lepers, returned a demoniac to sanity, took away Peter's mother-in-law's fever, healed a soldier's child and Jairus' daughter, and restored hearing to the deaf. These are just a few of his recorded greatest hits. On one day, the Bible tells us, "A huge crowd kept following him wherever he went because they saw his miraculous signs as he healed the sick" (John 6:2, NLT). Jesus constantly healed those in need.

Sometimes Jesus showed up personally. Other times, he healed from afar with a simple, spoken word. Sometimes his methods seemed bazaar.

In one of my favorite stories, Jesus heals a blind man in an unusual way. He asks the man if he wants his sight restored. The man answers, yes, of course. Jesus takes him by the hand, leads him out of town, spits on his eyes, and puts his hands on him. Jesus tells the man to open his eyes and see. The man says he sees people, but they look like trees walking around. Jesus puts his hands on the man's eyes again, and his sight is fully restored (Mark 8:22-26).

I enjoy pondering the point Jesus is making here. Is the message sometimes healing takes multiple attempts, healing doesn't usually happen the way you think it will, or Jesus uses the lowest things of the earth to divinely heal us? All those seem possible. *But, Lord, why spit?*

After his death, his disciples continued Jesus' healing ministry. The book of Acts records the growing number of people becoming believers of Jesus. The Biblical text paints a picture of the apostles performing an abundance of signs, wonders, and miracles. Huge crowds gathered, all hoping for healing. The Lord had apparently given Peter a double portion of the power to heal.

"In fact, when people knew Peter was going to walk by, they carried the sick out to the streets and laid them down on cots and mats, knowing the incredible power emanating from him would overshadow them *and heal them*. Great numbers of people swarmed into Jerusalem from the nearby villages. They brought with them the sick and those troubled by demons—and everyone was healed" (Acts 5:14-16, TPT).

Other versions of this passage seem to record Peter's physical shadow as having the power to heal. I generally don't like to stand in anyone's shadow. But I would have gladly stood in Peter's! Acts also bears witness to Peter having brought back to life Tabitha, a beloved woman of the city, who had gotten sick and died (See Acts 9:36-43, TPT).

Physical healing still occurs in the church today. I'll never forget the first experience of miraculous healing in which I had a part. A baby boy, only a few months old, in our congregation, was suffering from digestive problems. For unknown reasons, he had rejected breast milk and every possible baby formula. He cried all day and night in misery. Mom and Dad had no sleep. The doctors had no answers. Fearful for their baby's life, and desperate, they called me, their young and inexperienced pastor, to come to pray for his healing, lay hands on him, and anoint him with holy oil.

I came over quickly. In the family room, Mom, Dad, and I gathered around a sick baby boy. We all put our hands on him, taking turns praying. I prayed first with all my might, and then Dad prayed. Finally, Mom began to pray. When she did, the Spirit manifested in a special way, and she leaned in hard. It was like she took her baby in her arms and marched him up to the gates of heaven, where she pounded on the gates, begging God, demanding, and claiming mercy and healing in Jesus' name. When she finished, we stood in silence around the baby's crib, feeling his heart beating and listening to him breathe. Lastly, I marked a cross on his forehead with holy oil.

The next day, the mom called. "You won't believe this." After I had left, they fed their son a bottle of formula with no difficulty. After that, he slept all night. Praise the Lord! Since that night, he has not had any more problems eating or digesting food. God answered our prayers and healed him.

Over the passing years, I've seen other instances of healing. I've also seen times when the requested physical healing didn't come. In these disappointing and difficult times, God always seemed to provide healing in some other way.

We must acknowledge that there are many times when physical healing doesn't happen. We dare not offer false hope and empty platitudes. I can recall more times when physical healing didn't happen than when it did. I've witnessed people we prayed for die of ALS, CPOD, heart disease, and other diseases, as well as injuries from gunshots and car accidents and drug overdoses. I've watched newborn babies die. I've watched elderly patients die who'd suffered from Alzheimer's for years.

When I first heard Jesus tell me my illness would not end in death, that it was for the glory of God, I didn't want to tell anyone. Maybe because I wasn't totally sure I believed it myself. One reason that I kept my good news to myself was knowing so many people also believed in God's healing—many more faithful than I—but had not received it. I did not want my being healed to add to someone else's hurt.

Nonetheless, I know that physical healing can happen and does happen. If we have God, it is possible. We must believe it and should claim God's ability to do so. If God has in some way given you a special assurance that God plans to physically heal you, believe it with all your might. Don't let go for an instant.

Whether or not physical healing happens, God can and will heal in countless other ways. God can heal families, marriages, relationships, addictions, depression, loneliness, broken dreams, self-image, life-purpose, and more. I believe God can heal your country, community, church, company, and whatever else may be broken in your life.

As Christians, our ultimate and most crucial healing will occur when we have died and gone to heaven to be with God forever. Many times, our physical death is the most merciful healing possible and a gift. This is especially true if we die well— assured of God's love for us, filled with hope and the peace of Jesus, and at peace with one another, and most importantly, with God.

God is most concerned with our spiritual healing. Moreover, as we see in the following verse, our spiritual healing precedes other kinds of healing. "If my people, who are called by my name, will humble themselves and pray and seek my face and turn from their wicked ways, then I will hear from heaven, and I will forgive their sin and will heal their land" (2 Chronicles 7:14).

The healing God desires begins with healing our relationship with him. Through repentance, forgiveness, and prayer, our friendship with God can be restored. God also wants to "heal our land." That may mean favorable climate conditions and an abundant harvest, a healthy environment, protection from enemies, and general prosperity. It likely includes our relationship with the other people in our world, our nation, and our homes. God wants to heal the relationships of husband and wives, parents and children, siblings, and friends.

Jesus showed concern for the whole person, not just physical healing. He taught and showed people how to live in the Kingdom of God—how to have a relationship with God, each other, and the world. He provided food and healed hungry bellies, embraced the left-out and lonely and grafted them into

God's family, broke through racial divides, challenged abuse of power, and confronted those who loved wealth.

In the account of Jesus' sacrificial death on the cross, there is an example of Jesus' power to heal the brokenness in relationships that touches me. While hanging on the cross in incomprehensible agony, Jesus sees his mother, Mary. She is standing nearby, helplessly watching the gruesome and barbaric treatment of her son. John, one of Jesus' closest disciples and friends, stands beside Mary. Jesus sees them both and loves them both. In his pain, Jesus looks at his mom and somehow says, "Woman, here is your son." Then Jesus looks at John and says, "Here is your mother" (John 19:26-27).

God longs for our relationships with one another to be healed. That happens best, and perhaps only happens, when our relationship with God has been healed. The closer we grow to God, the closer we become to each other.

All of Jesus' miracles of physical healing demonstrate God's compassion for the hurting and those in need of healing. More importantly, they help us believe in and experience God's healing for ourselves.

If you look up *healing* in a Bible dictionary, you will find that healing can mean many things—therapy, the curing of disease, deliverance from what binds us, restoration of what's been lost, repairing of what's been broken, and in the broadest sense, salvation. Whatever word you prefer, all healing aims for the same outcome, God desires to make us holy and whole.

My cancer journey started with the revelation that I had a broken body. I wasn't as healthy and whole as I thought. Attending to the brokenness of my body brought into sight other areas of brokenness in my life. It was like going to see your doctor for one problem and finding out you have some other things wrong.

There was much more brokenness than I had imagined. I had brokenness in my relationships, brokenness in my sense of identity and broken trust. Each chapter of this book is about some place of brokenness in my life and how God brought healing into it. God used my cancer experience to reveal and heal all my brokenness.

Cancer added to my brokenness. Cancer broke my dreams and expectations for my future. My career as the church's pastor was finished. The actions of the church had broken my family's hearts. Their faith in the church, and maybe even God, had been dealt a severe blow. My trust in its leaders had been broken. Our plans for where we would live, all the exciting and wonderful things we looked forward to doing, had all been broken. The significant pay cut that came with medical leave, and the expense of moving, we feared would break the bank.

Nonetheless, through it all, I could see God picking up all the pieces of my broken life and creating a glorious mosaic. I had a new, promising chemotherapy drug, and I felt great. I loved having the time to write and be with my family. Amy and I were happier than ever. Our kids were thriving. I reconnected with friends. Lots of good things were happening. God was healing me, making me holy and whole again.

Physically, I felt good. Healing of the cancer continued. The number of tumors in my brain had shrunk. The new chemotherapy medication I had started didn't seem to be causing any problems. In my heart of hearts, I believed it would work.

By God's providence, Amy and I were having dinner with friends when one of them shared with us his experience of having been cured of Hepatitis C. A few years earlier his doctor had told him, "We are going to control your Hepatitis C for now, but soon we will cure it." As predicted, a couple of years later, the breakthrough happened, and his doctor called him with the good news. Within a couple of months of taking the medicine, he was cured of the disease, and his liver had started to heal itself.

Our friend's story encouraged me. His testimony came at just the right time, like a gift from God. I knew Hepatitis C wouldn't be the last disease cured. Cancer cures were being discovered and developed as we spoke. Many more were on the horizon. God would continue working through the medical community, inspiring and blessing their efforts. I could hear my oncologist one day saying to me, "We will control your cancer for now, but soon we will cure it."

I looked forward to the next scans and check-in. I could envision the cure. I believed the physical healing would continue.

I could also see God healing other brokenness in my life. I felt holy and whole in our new home. After the trauma of moving, we were getting settled. I could see God at work, healing our family. I felt joyful and strong. I felt more deeply connected and in love with Amy than ever. I enjoyed the time with our kids. I felt a greater appreciation for my family and friends and had more time to devote to them and spend with them. I felt joy, peace, and excitement as I continued writing and living into that calling.

We experienced healing in our finances. A few months after my diagnosis, Amy graduated from nursing school and landed a great job. With two incomes, soon, things were looking up financially. We were starting to dig ourselves out of the hole and were on our way to financial peace.

On the first day of medical leave, I received a generous grant from an agency of the Church to help us transition. A few days later, we received a check from my former congregation for a love offering they had taken up for us. The amount wildly surpassed our expectations. Let's just say it was "a whole lot of love."

Medical leave gave us access to some of the other significant financial resources we hadn't anticipated. One parishioner reached out and offered to pay the closing costs on our new home. Help came in many ways. Within a couple of weeks of medical leave, our bank balance was higher than it had ever been.

Deciding to cash in on this once-in-a-lifetime opportunity, we paid off most of our credit card debt. That eliminated several monthly payments from our budget, saving us money and making our financial life more comfortable and peaceful. We kept enough for our moving expenses and for a long weekend getaway we planned to take before our move date.

For the first time in as long as I could remember, we had financial peace. I stood in awe of how God had used cancer and medical leave to make us financially whole. Peace is the wholeness God's healing gives. I should have known and believed God would use the brokenness of cancer to help heal our financial brokenness.

On July 9, 2019, the morning of my almost two-year checkup with my oncologist, I woke up feeling unusually calm and optimistic—no "scanxiety" at all. Instead, I felt immense "scanticipation!" I believed *today could be the day*. I had been praying and knew others were, too, that I would hear the words, *The cancer is gone*. *The cancer has shrunk*, would be okay, but *The cancer is gone* would be great! I reminded myself and others of my most important prayer—that God would continue to be glorified through my illness.

It was like one of those rare days when everything seems to be going your way. The drive to the clinic, though longer from our new house, didn't feel longer. We arrived with thirty minutes to spare. Despite the parking deck bulging with vehicles, a spot opened for us as we made the first turn inside the deck. I didn't have to wait at any of the appointments. I'm not sure I even sat. The technicians I had for the MRI, CT Scan, and blood draw were all top tier. I got the A-team.

I felt energetic, healthy, and in good spirits as Amy and I sailed through the hospital from one appointment to the next. As we did, I thought, *I feel too good to be here. I don't belong here.*

We checked in for my appointment with my oncologist, and then joined my mom and dad in the waiting area. I filled out the intake form—no problems to report and zero distress. Check. Check. Check. I clipped the pen in place, set the clipboard down, and prepared to wait. My doctor seemed always to be running an hour or two late. The second the clipboard hit the table, my buzzer activated, indicating they were ready for me.

A few minutes later, my entourage and I were checked into the observation room and waiting for my oncologist. We had waited less than five minutes when the door opened, and a resident doctor entered the room. *Oh, Lord. Here we go with the practice round. I knew things were moving too fast to be true. I just want to see my doctor and get some results!*

The young doctor quickly introduced himself, took a seat, and got straight to the point. "I've got good news for you. They are all gone. All the tumors in your brain are gone."

We looked at each other in stunned silence, shocked by the young doc's abruptness and the awesomeness of the results. Without wasting any time, he showed us the images of my beautiful, cancer-free brain and lungs. He showed us the difference between these scans and the ones taken at my previous visit three months earlier. The contrast floored me—especially seeing my brain, peppered with little white spots only three months ago, now solid black.

We all grasped for words to express our joy. *Praise God! To God Be the Glory! That's amazing! How wonderful! Thank you, Jesus. I believed you!* I stood and hugged Amy. I wiped away the tears of joy. I hugged my mom and dad.

In our elation, Dr. Crawford entered and expanded on the good news. "The radiologists call this 'near-complete resolution of disease.' We are going to call these images *cancer-free*. Congratulations!"

As my Mom, Dad, Amy, and I sat overwhelmed with joy, holding hands and holding back tears, Amy sent out a flurry of texts updating friends and family. She showed me one of the elated responses, and I saw her original message, "NED cancer is gone!"

"Who's Ned?" I asked facetiously. "Are you talking to another man? Now?"

"No, silly. It's medical language. It means *no evidence of disease*."

"Oh, okay. I love Ned!"

That evening, we celebrated with family and friends at one of our favorite restaurants. After a beautiful, delicious dinner, friends revealed a cake upon which had been written, in icing, "NED Forever!"

On September 1st, 2017, I was diagnosed with stage four lung cancer. On July 9th, 2019, I was pronounced cancer-free. God had used cancer to cure me, and now God had cured my cancer. God had used the disease to bring healing into every part of my life. Now God had healed the disease. Thank you, God!

Glory

On July 9, 2019, after my doctor said the words, "No Evidence of Disease," and "cancer-free," we all looked for the right words. One word rose within the depths of my being, filled my heart and spirit, and poured forth from my lips. "Glory!"

Two years earlier, I had heard the Lord say to me, *This sickness will not end in death, but is for the glory of God and Jesus' glory* (John 11:4). A few days after that, the Lord reiterated his intentions: *You have cancer so that the mighty and glorious works of God can be displayed in your life* (John 9:3). These two promises guided my steps and gave me the strength to continue. I believed God's promise: "he who began a good work in you will carry it on to completion until the day of Christ Jesus" (Philippians 1:6).

God's glory had been on display in my life since my cancer diagnosis. God had used my cancer to bring healing into every part of my life. All of this had given me greater assurance that my physical healing would come. I recalled Jesus' challenge to the religious leaders who would not believe him when he told them he was the Son of God. "Even though you do not believe me, believe the works" (John 10:38). If I had ever not believed or doubted what Jesus had promised me, I had to believe him now because of his works in me.

God had healed me of cancer. That healing may have come because Jesus had commanded it on that day. God may have orchestrated my healing through his agents of science and medicine, over time. Maybe it was a combination. Either way, God had used the cancer to bring healing into every dimension of my life, and now God had healed me of the cancer. God had resoundingly demonstrated his power, love, and faithfulness. Only one word could adequately describe what had just happened—*glory!*

The day after my cancer-free appointment, the alarm clock sounded, and life resumed. I woke up wondering how I should feel after being healed and what I should do today. What should you do the day after being cured of cancer? Go to the gym and workout? Mow the grass? Lounge around the house in my pajamas? Should I plan a party to celebrate? Within a matter of minutes, Amy went back to work. The kids continued their summer sleep-ins. I fed the dogs and cats, made myself a cup of coffee, and sat to write. I wanted to be sure I captured the previous day's experience.

As I began to reflect, my mind turned to, of all things, pork chops. Growing up, one of the favorite meals my mom made for us regularly was something she called "glorified pork chops." Generally, pork chops are ordinary, plain. But that all changed when my mom added her glory sauce—a bright red, sweet, tangy concoction that made the pork chops look exceptional, even shine, and taste heavenly. It made everything on the plate taste delicious. My brothers and I poured it on our mash potatoes, like gravy, and dipped our green beans in it. I can hear my mom now: *"Don't lick your fingers, boys."*

When the doctors showed us the cancer-free scans, God poured glory sauce on my life. In the days to come, everything looked better and brighter. My neighborhood, the house, the pool, my family, my situation. It all tasted great. The Bible says, "O taste and see that the LORD is good" (Psalm 34:8, KJV). Everything seemed to shine and sparkle. Everything tasted sweeter.

I went to the grocery store to get some fruits for breakfast. The beauty of the apples struck me. They seemed to sparkle. The Golden Delicious looked delicious. The Gala apple's coloring looked like art. The strawberries seemed larger, shinier, and redder. I had never seen such a perfect tomato—big, red, firm, not a single bruise, bump, or scratch, and the perfect stem. Peppers—green, yellow, red, and orange—amazed me with their lines, curves, colors, and the curvature of the stem. The red onion looked like an artist had painted the purple peels. Even the bunches of lush green romaine lettuce shined as though they had come from the Garden of Eden.

As I walked home, the glorious weather elicited my praise. *Thank you, God, for these Carolina blue skies. Thank you for our neighborhood.* I marveled at it—beautiful, safe, and in a great location. I loved having sidewalks and looked forward to taking a dip in the community swimming pool.

I admired our house as I approached—two stories, with white siding and black trim. It stood, stately, at the corner, with a cute postage-stamp-sized yard, fenced-in backyard, and neat landscaping done by the previous homeowners. *Thank you very much, God.*

We missed our old house. It had been painful to leave such a grand home. We could never have afforded one like it on our own. Our new home was half the size of our old house. The rooms were much smaller, and there were fewer of them. Our new yard was cute, but tiny in comparison. The neighborhood wasn't as quiet. The bathrooms were smaller. In the master bathroom, you could sit on the tiny toilet and reach out and touch the tub. The location was convenient, but it wasn't Chapel Hill.

Nonetheless, it all looked perfect. The kitchen, the counters, the wall colors, the fixtures, the lighting, and even the hardware seemed nicer and more beautiful than anything we had ever had. We had miraculously gone from booger green linoleum counters to granite! And now we were cooking with gas. The hardwood floors seemed to shine. It wasn't as big, but it was everything we needed and more.

Our whole family loved the house from the moment we first walked into it. Just as I had all but given up on finding a house at all, God provided it like a gift from heaven.

After my first swim in the neighborhood pool, I sat at a table beside the pool, in a comfy chair under the oversized sun umbrella. I watched the parents playing with their children in the water, the sunbathers lounging around the deck, and the lifeguards in red trying to pay attention. With a cold drink in one hand and a tasty sandwich in the other, I felt like I was at a resort in the Caribbean. Delightfully amused and amazed, I smiled and asked myself, *Am I on medical leave, or is this a paid vacation?*

After lounging for a while and reading a book, I decided to swim a couple of laps. At the far end of the pool, I turned around to swim back. Before putting my head down into the water, I looked up at and saw the most picture-perfect scene. An array of sunbeams shone over the tree line and down at the water at just the right angle, making the surface sparkle and dance with light. The sun had moved, or a cloud had shifted in such a way as to allow the perfect amount of light through without blinding me, to create a dazzling and glorious light show to behold.

Not surprisingly, the Bible often likens God's glory to light. As I reflected, a few verses came to mind.

"The God who made light," the Apostle Paul proclaims, "lets his light shine in our hearts to give us the light of the knowledge of God's glory displayed in the face of Christ" (2 Corinthians 4:6).

"Let there be light!" God declared on day one of creation (Genesis 1:3). Before making anything else, God created light. Ever since, light has represented God and the things of God—love, life, truth, beauty, warmth, and more. Conversely, darkness often represents life without God.

To a world lost in the dark, Jesus says, "I am the light of the world. Whoever follows me will not walk in darkness but will have the light of life" (John 8:12, ESV). God's glorious light can shine through Jesus and into our lives. When that happens, we become like mirror balls, reflecting the glory light of God into the world.

The glory light helps us see the greatness and goodness of God. It makes us open our eyes. Its warmth draws us closer to God. Its illuminations reveal his presence in our lives. By it, we can see the wonders of God's creation. Light makes things shine, dazzle, and sparkle. It illuminates the truth of who we are, warts and all. But more importantly, it enables us to see who and what we can be.

I love the quote of C.S. Lewis that hangs on the wall of our living room. "I believe in the sun not because I can see it, but because by it I can see everything else."

Most of the time, sadly, we miss the glory. We don't taste the goodness of God. We don't see the sparkle and the brightness, maybe because we are too self-centered. Maybe because we are too distracted. Perhaps we have taken life for granted. Perhaps we have spent too much time in the darkness. I have certainly been guilty of each.

God used cancer to open my eyes to the glory all around me. I had seen a lot already. But the experience of receiving a cancer-free scan somehow switched on all the glory lights in the universe. I could see glory everywhere. I could join with the praise of the seraphim in Isaiah's vision of God. "Holy, holy, holy is the Lord Almighty; the whole earth is full of his glory" (Isaiah 6:3).

In the two years since my cancer diagnosis, I had gotten lots of tastes of the glory sauce. I had seen the bright light of God's glory shining over my life. At my one-year checkup, when doctors told me the tumor in my lung was gone, that was glorious. Philip's generosity glorified God in a special way. The change in my relationship with Amy had been glorious. There were glorious traces throughout my cancer journey.

But my physical healing topped them all. I had been baptized in the glory sauce. I had been dunked, immersed in it. I was swimming in it. Glory splashed over me. I had glory in my eyes. Everything seemed to sparkle and shine with God's glory.

After my cancer-free report, I desperately wanted to go worship at a church. I had gone a couple of times since leaving my job. The rest of the family preferred to stay home, but I felt a deep need to go. It didn't have to be a United Methodist Church. I just needed an opportunity to worship. I didn't feel any need to go based on allegiance or duty to anyone. I simply felt a genuine desire to give God thanks, praise, and glory.

I found a non-denominational church not far from my new house and went. I arrived at the church and found a parking lot full of parked cars and no human in sight. The church's doors were closed. No cars were coming or going. I rechecked the service time on the church's website. I had read it wrong. The service was almost halfway through.

I drove to a nearby United Methodist church only to find I had missed the worship service I would have attended. As I saw the worshippers starting to come out, I left and drove to another church a few minutes away. Its worship service had also looked interesting. I pulled into the parking lot, which also was fully packed with no person in sight, not even a greeter by the door. Another search confirmed my suspicion. Their service also was nearly over.

Sitting there feeling disappointed, I remembered that the first church I attempted had a second service that would start thirty minutes after the first service. I decided to go back where I'd started, slip in for the second half of the first service, and then stay for the first half of the next service. One way or the other, I was going to worship!

The pastor preached an excellent sermon, which ended the first service. During the break between services, a few people spoke to me. Mostly, I enjoyed having the time to be quiet and sit in the sanctuary. The large traditional sanctuary with cushioned pews, stained glass windows, and a baptistry had been reclaimed for a modern service. Two large screens at the front on both the left and right sides displayed church announcements, and later, words to the songs we would sing. At center stage, a microphone and acoustic guitar awaited the worship leader. On the right side, I could see the keyboard and a drum set. On the left side, the bass guitar and electric guitar stood waiting.

The room darkened as the service started. The band took the stage and started playing. The worship leader enthusiastically welcomed everyone and invited us all to stand, sing, and worship. I liked him. The band sounded great. I loved the songs and could sing them all, even the one new to me by Elevation Worship, one of my favorite worship bands. The lyrics about God accomplishing whatever he says and always keeping his promises spoke to me deeply.

The twenty or thirty people attending the service were able to spread out in the large sanctuary. The house lights were turned off, creating a dark and intimate experience, which I appreciated. As we sang, I raised my open hands. I followed the worship leader through the next two songs. I stuck my arms straight up overhead. I pumped my arms up and down. "Yes, God. Thank you, Jesus." I loved the band's high energy. I clapped. I shouted, "Amen!" I sang my heart and lungs out. I worshipped and praised God with all my being. I loved every second of it.

Just when I thought the glorious service couldn't get any better, the worship leader started strumming his acoustic guitar and signaled to the other musicians to stop as he started singing the old hymn "Great is Thy Faithfulness."[11] When we got to the chorus, I had begun to dissolve into tears and could only mouth the words:

"Great is Thy faithfulness."
Morning by morning, new mercies I see.
All I have needed Thy hand hath provided.
"Great is thy faithfulness," Lord, unto me!

I felt gratitude, humility, and awe. By the time we reached the last verse and sang about God providing "strength for today and bright hope for tomorrow," I was a snotty mess, shaking all over and thanking God for the darkness that hid me. I somehow pulled myself together as the song ended. While the pastor gave the final benediction, I dried my eyes and face. By the time the technician raised the house lights, I was presentable.

With that, the first half of the service concluded, and I slipped out. After two half-services, I left with one full heart.

For our family's summer beach trip, we returned to the beachfront condo I enjoyed alone at the first of the year. This time, we filled it with family, friends, and love for one another.

We spent the week on the beach, swimming and splashing in the ocean and sunbathing and walking on the sandy shore. We stood in awe of the beauty of creation. We read and listened to music. Wannabe mixologists made piña coladas and margaritas and sent relief from the cottage to the sunbathers.

In our cottage by the sea, we sat on the porch and delighted in the breeze, listened to the ocean sounds, and gazed on the horizon. Weary puzzlers pieced together thousand-piece puzzles. Hungry beach bums snacked and munched. We prepared meals together and feasted. We danced to our favorite songs.

Once or twice, we left the condo for a round of mini-golf and to explore nearby shops and restaurants. We celebrated Amy's birthday at a fancy restaurant, and afterward had a picture of us all taken on the rooftop bar, with the ocean at our backs.

All of this we had done before on many family beach trips. But this time, it all seemed more special, wonderful, beautiful, joyful, and brighter. This beach trip, at least for me, was the most glorious of them all.

After my cancer-free report, I could see God's glory in my children more than ever. I could see it in Hannah, when she sang in her performances, when she advocated for justice, and as she prepared for her first year of college. I saw the sparkle, the glory in Marcie, as she told us about her new apartment and roommate, the teaching classes she planned to take, and her sorority. I saw the glory of God in Caleb, when he played guitar or piano and sang, as he played sports, and as he made new friends and got ready for his first year of high school.

I could surely see God's glory in Amy. The Bible says, "A good woman is hard to find and worth far more than diamonds" (Proverbs 31:10). She sparkled like a diamond. God's glory reflected off all her sides and even the edges. To know God handcrafted her to be my partner made her shine even more brightly. All that I loved about her—beauty, strength, determination, knowledge, loyalty, fierce love, and much more—manifested the glory of God.

After my cancer-free report, everything seemed brighter and more marvelous and important. Jesus had said that once he was glorified, God's glory would be on display, and there would be "glory all around" (John 13:31-32, Message). Now, with so many displays of God's holiness in my life, so much glory sauce, and glory light, there truly was glory all around.

"To God be the glory forever and ever. Amen"

—(Galatians 1:5, GNT).

Epilogue

Upon the completion of *How Cancer Cured Me*, we continue to reside in Raleigh, North Carolina. Our children are thriving—two in college, one in high school. Amy continues to excel as a registered nurse at Duke Hospital. Our marriage is still going strong, and I'm still getting good reports from my doctors. Life is good.

Clinically speaking, there continues to be no evidence of disease. Thank God for NED! I hope for the day when doctors tell me I'm permanently, once and for all, cured of cancer. I long to see a medication developed that can deliver that promise. Until then, I will continue to take the cancer-inhibiting chemotherapy drugs, to have my quarterly regime of scans and appointments, and hope to keep hearing the words *cancer-free*.

Spiritually speaking, I consider myself physically healed by Jesus. I believe he has used my cancer to cure me and cured me of cancer. That's what the Great Physician told me, and I'm sticking with that. At the beginning of my cancer journey, God promised to heal me. On July 9, 2019, God fulfilled his promise to me. Now the challenge is to have enough faith to continue to believe this healing is for life. God will not pull the rug out from under me. The scans and oncology appointments, daily medications, and even the side effects will be for me a constant reminder of how God healed me of cancer **and** used cancer to cure me.

It is important for me to confess, and for the reader to understand that the work God has begun in me continues. I am a very long way from sainthood. Every facet of the healing God accomplished in my life from my diagnosis to my first cancer-free report continues to this day. I continue to strive to become more patient, forgiving, courageous, and all the rest. The changes I have recorded in this book are real, and often dramatic, but they are not yet complete. God continues to use my cancer experience to help me become the person he created me to be.

I do not know now what the future holds for me in terms of pastoral leadership in a church setting. I continue to heal and to discern God's plan for my family and me. Whatever that may be, I know it will be good.

I still feel called to ministry, and many have continued to affirm that for me. After I preached the sermon at my father-in-law's funeral, my dad found me in the church's atrium and made a beeline towards me, mouthing, *"Great job!"* on his approach. He hugged me, kissed me on the head, and whispered in my ear, "Remember your calling. Remember your calling." Never had I received such loving affirmation from my dad. It is worth more to me than all the riches in the world.

I will continue to write. One of the blessings of writing this book, along with all the journaling and blogging, has been the rediscovery of how much I love to write. When I was just learning my letters, on a little scrap piece of paper, I wrote, "I am a writer," for my mom to read. I believe God created me to write. Writing was always one of my favorite and most celebrated parts of my ministry in the church, but one I could devote limited time to. I hope to continue to devote substantial time and energy to writing. Writing may provide me a larger platform for preaching and teaching the good news of Jesus Christ.

I feel a calling to continue writing materials that can minister to those living with or impacted by cancer. In addition to working hard to promote *How Cancer Cured Me*, I will continue to write about the limitless ways God can use cancer for good and heal our cancer. I want to help those experiencing cancer to know and draw near to Jesus Christ and experience God's transforming love.

I recently launched a website, www.davidgira.com. Please visit me at my online home. I will continue to share blog posts, devotions, reflections, and other materials that I hope can help others connect with Christ. God is present and can and will bless the best and the mess. God can use our brokenness to heal us and heal our brokenness. His mighty works and glory are always on display. We simply need help opening our eyes, seeing what is before us, and hearing the word of the Lord.

I want all my writing and ministry, in whatever form they take, to open eyes and hearts to the love of God through faith in Jesus Christ. The greatest work of all is helping others grow in a living, loving, spirit-filled relationship with God through Jesus. Nothing is more important to me. In that sense, I will always be a pastor. In all that I write, I want to point readers to Jesus Christ as Savior and Lord and help them take steps in his direction. The healing we need, everything we need is found in Jesus.

Endnotes

1   "Lung Cancer Facts." Lung Cancer Initiative, www.lungcancerinitiativenc.org/lung-cancer-facts.

2   "A Charlie Brown Christmas," written and created by Charles M. Schulz (1965; Hollywood, California: Paramount Pictures, 2000), DVD.

3   "Distinctive Wesleyan Emphases." The United Methodist Church, November 6, 2013. https://www.umc.org/en/content/distinctive-wesleyan-emphases.

4   Seuss. *How the Grinch Stole Christmas*. New York: Random House, 1957.

5   Piper, Watty. *The Little Engine That Could*. New York : Philomel Books : in association with Grosset & Dunlap, 2005.

6   Wesley, Charles "Come, Thou Long Expected Jesus", 1744.

7   Heschel, Abraham Joshua. *The Sabbath*. (New York: Farrar, Straus and Giroux, 1975), 18.

8   Ibid, 19.

9   Foster, Richard J. *Celebration of Discipline: the Path to Spiritual Growth*. (San Francisco: HarperSanFrancisco, 1998), 172.

10 Tidying Up with Marie Kondo. "Tidying with Toddlers." Season 1, Episode 1. Netflix, March 14, 2020.

11 Chisholm, Thomas O. *Great Is Thy Faithfulness*. Music by William M. Runyan. (Chicago: Hope Publishing Company, 1923).

About the Author

David Gira graduated from Duke University's Divinity School in 2005, where he received his Master of Divinity with honors. He is an ordained elder of the United Methodist Church and member of the North Carolina Annual Conference. He has eighteen years of pastoral and church leadership experience. Since being diagnosed with stage 4 lung cancer in 2017, he has devoted his ministry to supporting cancer patients and their loved ones. He is a frequent blogger and now a published author. He and his wife Amy have been married for twenty-three years and have three children. They currently reside in Raleigh, North Carolina.

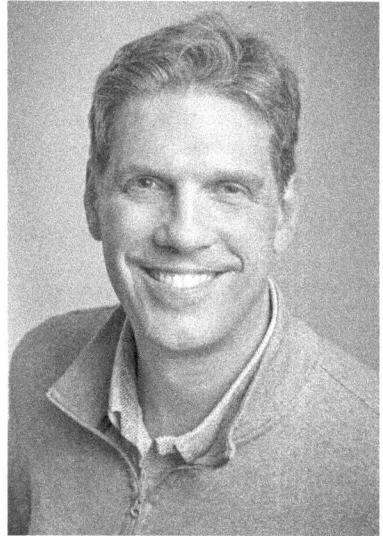

www.ingramcontent.com/pod-product-compliance
Lightning Source LLC
Chambersburg PA
CBHW030829090426
42737CB00009B/933